NATURALLY

THIN

A Blueprint to Stay Thin

And Healthy ALWAYS!

By Dr. Rafael Bolio

TITLE: NATURALLY THIN: A blueprint to stay thin and healthy ALWAYS

AUTHOR: DR. RAFAEL BOLIO

FIRST EDITION JANUARY 2018

Library of Congress Control Number: TXu 2-058-286

Printed in the United States of America

ISBN 978-0-9997799-0-3 (paperback)

ABOUT THE BOOK COVER: the Leonardo da Vinci Vitruvian man demonstrates the blend of mathematics and art and Leonardo's deep understanding of proportions. It is a representation of perfect health. Since this book is based on the proportions theory and strives to obtain perfect health, I have used the image to illustrate my program.

Dr. Rafael Bolio.

Disclaimer: this book contains advice and information related to the accumulation of excess body fat. It does not replace the advice of a doctor or another trained health professional. Dr. Bolio is a doctor and a specialist in Internal Medicine in his native country. However, he is not giving medical advice or diagnosis. The contents of this book cannot be used to diagnose, prevent, or treat any disease. In the event you use any of the information of this book, the author assumes no responsibility for your actions.

--CONTENTS--

To my brother Ruvince, in memory,

To My Children

To Deborah,
who taught me how to write in English.

To all my patients,
who believed in me even when I didn't.

DIRTY WORDS

You are being warned!

This book will have many dirty words, and I hope that you will bear with me in my use of these words. It is not that I purposefully want to be rude, it is just that many of these words have now become incredibly emotionally charged!

So, I am going to start with the first dirty four-letter word:

DIET

Ugh!

I also want to add to the list the word OBESITY and OBESE, which will occasionally be used. These words do not seem to be politically correct nowadays, although they were certainly quite normal years ago. I have changed these dirty words into a new set of words: "excess body fat". But for clarity's sake, when necessary, I will use OBESITY and OBESE, ok?

And then there are the other ugly words: fat, overweight, thin, excess weight, etc., etc.

If you find other words that make you uncomfortable, please forgive me in advance, and again, bear in mind that I am not trying to be insulting just to grab your attention.

This a workbook with information as well as philosophy.

If you want to start the diet immediately, go straight to Week 1 on page 41.

Once you have finished this week, go back and read READY, SET, GO! starting on page 37. This chapter explains what will be happening to your body in the following weeks, and it is very important to know what to expect.

From there you should advance to read and apply WEEK 2, 3, 4, etc.

Now, if you want to have a broader outline of what this book is about, first read THE ADIPOSE SYSTEM which starts on page 7.

If you want to find out how just how savvy you are regarding excess body fat and its treatment, just do the test in FINDING YOUR LIFE PARTNER on page 11.

If you want some fabulous tips to get the best results out of this and any other diet, read GETTING BETTER RESULTS which starts on page 33.

If you want to obtain targeted fat loss and body shaping, first read THE OBESITY SISTERS starting on page 23. After that, read FOR DOCTORS AND NUTRITIONISTS on page 152 where the mathematical equations used for targeted fat loss are outlined.

And then comes the best part of all, which is keeping excess body fat off!

To do that, **READ ALL THE BOOK**!

THERE IS NO WAY AROUND IT.

You must read the whole book so that the lifetime program makes sense, and most important so that you are successful in staying thin for the rest of your life!

Oh, and ideally you should read the whole book at least three times.

And don't you dare lend this book to anyone, because it will never come back. Tell your friends to buy their copy!

Happy hunting!

THE ADIPOSE SYSTEM

OK, so you're not a doctor or nutritionist, but still want to read the first three chapters of this book, which are all about theory. That's fine; just don't worry if some of the terms seem complicated or difficult to understand.

Now, if you're the type of person who wants to solve the problem YESTERDAY, go straight to the diet on WEEK ONE on page 41. However, I earnestly invite you to come back and carefully read the book from beginning to end, at least three times.

This way, you will understand why we will be doing things the way we are.

Here we go.

With all the current information we have, it should be easy to help people lose their excess fat permanently, right?

Wrong.

If we want to treat excess body fat successfully, we must first understand that it is a system, just like the immune system, the cardiovascular system, or the central nervous system.

I propose that we call it the ADIPOSE SYSTEM.

THE ADIPOSE SYSTEM

So, have we discovered a new system? Of course not! It's been right under our noses, but we just weren't paying attention to it until it started becoming a "huge" problem. It is "weighing" heavily on the health system, it "burdens" down self-esteem, and it is a "heavy load" to bear!

The adipose system interconnects with every other system of the body, especially the immune system.

Both the adipose system and immune system respond at the same time. Such is the case with excess body fat and rheumatoid arthritis and asthma. What's even more interesting is that both work in tandem.

Why do we need the adipose system?

That one is easy; we need it to defend our bodies just like the immune system.

And how does the adipose system defend us?

It protects our body by storing nutrients for when there is an increased need for them.

We used to think that the only activity of the adipose system was to store and release fat, but we were wrong.

When the body needs it, it will use up the whole adipose cell to obtain whatever is required for survival. You read it right, we can cannibalize our own fat cells!

There's plenty of evidence to prove that.

Just check what happens with the HCG (human chorionic gonadotropin) protocol, where you are using a disastrously restricted unbalanced diet, and despite this, there are no signs of sagging skin, nor loss of breast firmness, falling hair, or vitamin deficiencies. Where does the body get what it's not receiving from the diet? My guess is that we obtain it from the whole adipose cell.

And then there's my juicing diet which INCREASES breast size in women and at the same eliminates waistline. How can the body cause that when it is only receiving 1,300 calories per day? By using the whole adipose cell.

There's also research as to how different phytochemicals block circulation to the fat cell without any signs of necrosis. How in the world does that happen?

It will take some time to find the perfect combination of nutrients and perhaps medications to increase the body's ability to use up its fat cells without generating Starvation Mode. The possibility is there, but we must stop thinking about restrictions and start thinking about the right ingredients.

Now if we describe what it defends us from, then things get really complicated and fascinating.

Think about it, not only is it protecting us from physical aggression, but it also protects us from abstract aggressions like fear, hatred, anxiety, etc.

Do you want to see a clear connection between thoughts and the body? Just study the adipose system.

One last comment. If you want plenty of stem cells, you are going to get them in the adipose system. They work in tandem with the adipose system's reserve and recovery function that makes us a spectacular survival machine.

It is truly a fascinating system.

Think about this; we would have perished thousands of years ago from famine and disease without the adipose system. If there was a monument created to honor humanity's greatest gift from nature, it should be the adipose cell.

We need to view the adipose system with the utmost respect, just like all the other systems. And we need to teach our patients to do the same.

We can divide fat in our body into two compartments, structural fat, and the adipose system.

We do not want to get rid of structural fat, nor should we.

We do not want to get rid of 80% of our brain, or a third of every cell membrane wall, or pericardium, or mesentery, or breasts, or gluteal fat, or hormones, or prostaglandins, etc., etc., etc.

Perhaps tomorrow, we will discover that there is a disease that arises from structural fat, but even then, we certainly will not want to eliminate it.

The other one, the one we all hate to have, is the adipose system, the one that accumulates inside the abdomen, under the skin, and in almost every other part of our body.

Excess body fat is the fat that we must regulate.

But we must change all the terrible misinformation that there is about the adipose system.

First, we do not want to ELIMINATE the adipose system. We can't. It would be like trying to remove the cardiovascular system.

When the immune system fails, we do not want to get rid of it; we want to regulate it.

I have always viewed excess weight as a sign, just like a fever. It is a sign of something else going on wrong.

Although we treat the fever when it is excessive, we certainly do not believe that all is well with our patients by just giving them an aspirin.

If this were the solution, we would not need antibiotics, antivirals, cancer drugs, immune regulators, or even doctors.

If we do not address the cause of fever, all hell can break loose.

So that's what we do as doctors, we try to discover just what is causing that illness, and if needed, work tirelessly to help the body solve it.

We have gone dead wrong in the way we treat the adipose system's response. We are focusing on the sign and not the cause of that sign. We are treating weight gain and not the cause of weight gain.

So, let's find out just how much you know about why the adipose system kicks in and about how you can permanently eliminate excess body fat, ok?

I hope that the test in the next chapter will be fun, and most importantly, eye-opening!

FINDING YOUR LIFE PARTNER

In matrimony as well as in diets, we must be cautious in choosing the right partner with whom we will spend the rest of your lives. We certainly don't want to end up divorced and so bitter that we decide never to remarry or worse still, live our lives in pain and misery with the wrong spouse or bad diet.

Similarly, you don't want to go on a diet that makes you suffer all day, or that is so boring that you want to cheat on it all the time or become so frustrated with results that it makes you never want to diet again!

With a problem as complex and challenging as excess body fat and its treatment, it's well worth knowing what we are getting into and why we are doing it, or we may worsen a problem instead of solving it.

If you have been on a diet, are planning to go on a diet, want to avoid gaining weight, or even if you'd just like to help someone else lose weight, please take the following quiz to find out just how up to date you are on why you gain excess body fat. And most important, to see how much you know about new weight loss strategies:

Eating large quantities of rice generates excess fat:

TRUE _____ FALSE _____

Eating small frequent meals makes you thin:

TRUE _____ FALSE _____

The more raw almonds you eat, the more you gain weight:

TRUE _____ FALSE _____

Overweight people are less active than thin people:

TRUE _____ FALSE _____

I should feel guilty when I eat food that can make me fat:

TRUE _____ FALSE _____

Eating pasta for dinner makes me thin:

TRUE _____ FALSE _____

I should feel afraid of eating certain food:

TRUE _____ FALSE _____

Overweight people have weak will power:

TRUE _____ FALSE _____

Eating as much as you want makes you thin:

TRUE _____ FALSE _____

Strict diets worsen my excess body fat:

TRUE _____ FALSE _____

Now, let's look at the correct answers:

Eating large quantities of rice generates excess fat: FALSE

Those who still believe that carbohydrates such as rice make you fat have not read a timeworn prestigious medical journal published in January 1989: The Medical Clinics of North America. I suspect that the Chinese living in China have carefully read this document since the base of their diet is rice, they eat over 3,000 calories a day, and very few of them have excess fat. Carbohydrates will help you lose excess fat. The solution is simple; we must learn how to eat them correctly to get thin.

Eating small frequent meals makes you thin: FALSE

Talk about investigators going back and forth! First, we were told three meals a day, then we were told to eat five small meals per day, but recent research has found that five small meals will not help you lose weight if you are choosing the wrong meals! Again, being thin is not about eating many times a day; it is about knowing what to eat and when to eat it.

The more raw almonds you eat, the more you gain weight: FALSE

Information is quickly changing, and foods that were once thought to cause overweight are now turning out to be some of the best ways of treating it. One of these highly and wrongly slandered food groups is seed such as almonds, pecans, pistachios, etc. Recent research has shown that not only can they be eaten raw without gaining weight; they can even help you lose excess pounds and inches.

Overweight people are less active than thin people: FALSE

Due to the load generated by excess body fat, a person with excess weight who walks needs as much energy as a thin person who runs. Overweight individuals move less, but that movement requires greater energy. They are as active or even more than a thin person.

I should feel guilty when I eat food that can make me fat: FALSE

Again of excess fat is often associated with poor eating habits and has nothing to do with moral values. Virtue or loyalty is not in play when we have the dilemma of eating, or not eating a chocolate cake.

Chocolate cakes were made to be enjoyed and not to generate an "existential crisis." If you have a deep and dark psychological need to go have an "existential crisis" with pastry, go ahead and eat it anyway.

Eating pasta for dinner makes me thin: TRUE

Pasta is the Italian version of rice (see the answer to question number 1). If used correctly, pasta can be a fantastic weight loss tool.

I should feel afraid of eating certain food: FALSE

Hey, guys, we don't run on electricity or gasoline, we run on food! So why should we do it with fear? Fear of foods only causes confusion in the minds of people who diet (or those who want to avoid gaining weight), and as you will discover later in the book, it makes you gain even more excess fat!

Overweight people have weak willpower: FALSE

There is nothing more messed up than this idea about the treatment of excess body fat. What we need is a beautiful and sensible program that we can turn into a lifestyle. Would you need willpower if you are madly in love with your weight loss program? I don't think so.

Eating as much as you want makes you thin: TRUE

Once you learn the right way to eat any food in the amount you want, you will notice that excess body fat will slowly disappear. It is possible – and even necessary – to eat until you are satisfied to eliminate excess body fat.

Strict diets worsen excess body fat: TRUE

Strict diets will make you fatter. I was the first author to report that under-nutrition/ malnutrition generated excess body fat. Numerous researchers have now corroborated this phenomenon.

Why does severe dieting cause a greater accumulation of body fat?

Our body protects itself against restricted food intake by a series of adaptations known as Starvation Mode. For millennia, we have had to cope with a lack of nutritious and/or balanced foods.

To survive in regions where food was scarce, we developed this extraordinary defense mechanism. Starvation Mode is triggered when food intake is reduced or altered, and it is the reason why people regain their previous weight when they stop their weight loss program.

What's your score?

Add up all correct answers and write down the total: _____. Now, let's interpret your results:

Interpretation

7 to 10:   Excellent!

You are up to date as to why your body stores excess fat. If you are overweight, it probably is due to the inappropriate application of your nutritional program. I call these people the Illustrated Obese!

4 to 6:   You're going down the wrong path!

You have filled your mind with myths about why you accumulate excess body fat. These false ideas are interfering with your attempts to solve it.

3 or less: Way off base!

Besides lacking adequate information, you are living a series of emotional reactions that limit your recovery. You must re-learn to intensely enjoy all types of foods, including those that have been demonstrated to be associated with accumulation of excess body fat.

If your score is less than seven, don't worry about it. Many who take this quiz – including those who have been dieting all their lives – get a very low score.

What is cause for concern is not the prevalence of low scores, but the fact that so many go on diets without understanding why they gain excess body fat and, most important, oblivious to the fact that the wrong diet can cause major damage… and even more weight gain!

Why is there so much confusion surrounding this issue?

Excess body fat is one of the most complex phenomena in nature. It has baffled even the most brilliant researchers. Here is only one little tidbit of information that can make you dizzy: depending on circumstances, eating lettuce can make you either gain or lose excess body fat! Talk about complicated!

Obesity research is so complex that it causes many misinterpretations. Here are some common faulty assumptions:

If you eat fewer carbs or sugars (sugar, honey, jam, quinoa, bread, rice, pasta, fruit, etc.), you will lose weight and inches. Therefore, eating carbs causes excess body fat.

Answer: False

When you cut down animal protein (meat, chicken, fish, etc.), you lose weight and inches. It means that excess body fat is the result of eating animal protein.

Answer: False

If you go on a fat-free diet (no avocado, butter, cream, etc.), you lose weight and inches. Therefore, eating fat causes excess body fat.

Answer: False

A great reason for misunderstandings is that people wrongly consider that weight loss is equal to becoming naturally thin.

However, …

Losing weight is not the same as becoming naturally thin!

Metaphorically speaking, we are in the Dark Ages of weight loss:

During thousands of years, people were sure that the sun circled the earth because that is what THEY SAW. The information seemed unequivocal until someone came along and said, "we had it all wrong, it turns out that the earth circles the sun."

The fact that you lose weight when you don't eat carbs or reduce calories does not mean that carbs or calories are the cause of excess body fat, just like the sun rising in the east and setting in the west does not mean that it spins around the earth. Things are way, way more complicated.

Think about it: taking aspirin will make the fever go away, but it doesn't treat any underlying infection. Likewise, going on a strict diet makes you lose weight, but it does not generate a permanent fat loss.

Heck, you might even obtain a low weight with a strict diet and STILL HAVE EXCESS BODY FAT! Read again: having a normal weight is no guarantee that you have normal body fat.

There is a world of difference between losing weight (seeing changes on the scale) and becoming naturally thin (having healthy body fat without dieting).

You can lose weight by cutting sugars (bread, beans, fruit, etc.), fats, (avocado, butter, etc.), proteins (meat, fish, etc.), or all three. You can also achieve it by taking drugs like amphetamines, thyroid hormones, and diuretics. Severe diabetes, AIDS, some types of cancer, and many other diseases also make you lose weight.

This weight loss has nothing to do with becoming naturally thin since once the illness goes away or is controlled (or the drug is suspended, or the diet is abandoned), excess boy fat will return. None of these circumstances will make a fat person naturally thin. Naturally thin people don't diet, don't take weight loss pills, or exercise, or need to have cancer to stay thin.

If you didn't catch it, let me repeat it again: NATURALLY THIN PEOPLE DON'T DIET.

To be naturally thin, you must do what naturally thin people do: eat as much as you want of all food groups!

Many have spent their lives trying to lose weight (as opposed to becoming naturally thin) with the false hope that whatever they are doing will "fix" their metabolism. However, when you reduce or stop your food intake, it's impossible to "fix" your metabolism.

When you severely restrict your nutrient intake long enough, Starvation Mode is triggered, and that is why you regain excess weight. Diets only make you lose weight for a while.

To become permanently thin, you must eat like a naturally thin person!

At a conference of the North American Association for the Study of Excess body fat (NASO) in 1997, the experts concluded that due to the dramatic metabolic changes caused by limiting food intake, there were no diets, medications, or surgical procedures that permanently eliminate excess body fat. Years have passed, and this sad situation has not changed.

So, how do you know if you've become naturally thin, or have only lost weight?

Just answer this question: are you still dieting?

If the answer is YES, then you are not a naturally thin person.

If you regained any of the weight you lost (or have gained even more), it means that you are still in trouble. You did not achieve your desire to become naturally thin.

The only option for eliminating excess body fat for good is to change "fat behavior" for "thin behavior."

We must define excess body fat regarding behavior as well as percentages (over 30% of body fat in women and over 25% of body fat in men).

My obesity classification adds the following behavioral definitions:

Evident obese

Obese disguised in a thin body

Enlightened obese

Naturally thin people

Evident obese: the mirror will tell them that they have excess body fat (over 25% or 30%, depending on sex). Regarding behavior, most eat with fear and guilt; they obsess over their weight; dislike or hate their bodies; may have low self-esteem and above all have fat-generating habits that increase fat accumulation (i.e. they diet). They are fat, inside and out.

Obese disguised in a thin body: these people have a healthy weight, or may even be underweight. Heck, they might even look spectacular! However, they maintain their figures through diet, exercise, medications, body wraps, etc. Neither bulimics (those who vomit what they eat) nor anorexics (those who eat very little), or people who maintain their weight with diets can be classified as naturally thin people because while they are indeed thin, their behavior is not natural, and they practice eating habits just like the Evident Obese. They are thin on the outside and fat on the inside.

Enlightened obese: they are people from previous categories on the road to recovery: they have lost their fear of food, do not feel guilty after eating anything, accept their bodies and have high self-esteem. They have changed their fattening eating habits for naturally thin eating habits and know that sooner or later, they will get rid of their excess fat. They are fat on the outside, but thin on the inside.

Naturally thin people eat without fear or guilt. They don't need to diet, exercise, take medications, or use body wraps to be thin. They have slender bodies due to their eating habits. They are thin inside and out.

In this book, I'll show you how to become naturally thin by changing behavior to lose weight. I want you to stop being an evident obese, or an obese disguised in a thin body.

Becoming naturally thin requires patience and prudence. You will discover how to get thin by eating as much as you want of all food groups, but be aware that it requires discipline. You will learn how to eat everything to get thin. It's challenging, but many people have already succeeded!

What are the differences between a program that helps you get thin, and a program that just makes you lose weight?

Here are just a few rules for a program that helps you get naturally thin:

1. It includes all food groups. If programs promise you they will cure you, but limit the intake of some food group or all your food, they're lying to you. Restrictions will only cause you to lose weight.

2. It allows you to eat enough to feel satisfied, any time of day. The idea is to eat to become thin.

3. It allows you to enjoy food! In addition to being essential for survival, food has the significant advantage of providing pleasure. Every time you eat, especially if your body requires it, you experience an intense sensation of well-being. It is due, in part, to your body releasing substances known as endorphins. If a program is pleasurable, that's one more reason to stick with it. Pleasure helps you stay with your diet on the long term, which contributes to permanent weight loss.

4. The focus is not on weight. When a program insists that the most important point is weight loss, it's because it's not going to change your habits for those of a thin person. Weight is the least critical element when eliminating excess body fat. Unfortunately, people focus on the scale because they don't know how to become naturally thin!

5. It is slow but permanent. An increase in body fat causes a series of metabolic changes. Spectacular reductions of weight and volume don't give the body time to correct these changes. That's one of the many reasons why weight comes back. You need time to recover normal chemical processes. Our metabolism could care less about emotional needs to lose weight quickly. If you stress your body with strict diets, body, mind, and soul will all be undesirably affected.

6. It incorporates behavioral changes. A piece of pastry can make you thin or fat, depending on how you eat it. You will confirm this once you have used the program and reduced your body fat with pastry.

7. It doesn't need exercise, massages, supplements, or any magical product. If the program uses anything extra or different from food, then it's only a weight loss program and not a strategy to change you into a naturally thin person.

Don't get me wrong: I am not against exercise, massages or supplements. They can have a place in our daily life, but not in helping us change the way we eat.

According to results obtained in workshops I created, people show positive, spontaneous habit changes after just four weeks. They clearly identified what, when and how much to eat, and two things happen spontaneously: they chose fewer fat-filled foods and ate more fruits and vegetables.

Habit changes (engaging in a repetitive behavior unconsciously and efficiently) occurred 12 weeks into the program. From then on, "eating thin" became a natural response.

How can YOU learn to "eat to be naturally thin"?

I have come up with different options.

My first one was through the book Diets Make You Fat – Eating Makes You Thin, which gives a series of menus that help people prove to themselves that they can, in fact, "eat anything to be thin."

It has generated spectacular bodies in thousands of people who are to this day, still naturally thin. It's even read in schools of nutrition when studying treatments of excess body fat.

But there is a catch: for it to work, people must eat what is written in the amounts it says, even when they can eat more and still lose excess fat.

Individuals who don't like the recommendations, or are intolerant to gluten, or afraid of them are out of luck.

The book Diets Make You Fat – Eating Makes You Thin does not give the option of eating differently from what is on the menu.

This new book fills a gap that the previous one left since you will have dozens of choices to help you prepare the menu that best suits you.

If you're looking for a rapid loss of weight and measurements through a program that shows you exactly what to do, the book Diets Make You Fat – Eating Makes You Thin provides you with the results you want.

In this book, you will use a rigid menu that becomes more and more flexible and varied as the weeks advance. You will get to the point where you know how to balance almost every meal you can think of.

The logical long-term way to lose excess body fat is to change your current eating habits for those of naturally thin people.

You must stop dieting in the traditional sense of calorie restriction.

And you do have to learn how to balance all food groups in enough quantities to avoid at all cost Starvation Mode.

To achieve a permanent solution, you must change your eating behavior, instead of eating less or not eating at all.

In other words, you simply must learn how to eat to be thin!

But before we dive into the program I would like to answer the next question:

Why is it that we get fat?

This answer is quite fascinating, and I hope you thoroughly enjoy this next chapter which should be quite educational!

You might even end up furious for not having anyone give you this information before.

But just be careful, because anger makes you fat!

So, let's find out why the body accumulates excess body fat.

THE OBESITY SISTERS

As far as science has defined when and why our body accumulates fat, there are four primary reasons:

MALNUTRITION/UNDERNUTRITION
OVERNUTRITION
PROLONGED AND FREQUENT FASTING
STRESS

I will add two more categories:

LOW-CALORIE INTAKE
NEO-FORMATIONS

This classification leads us to ask if they all show up in the body in the same way.

It would make no sense since on one side fat is stored because of eating less and on the other because of overeating.

After measuring bodies of hundreds and hundreds of patients on a diet, I realized that in effect, fat is eliminated in entirely different areas.

Therefore, I call them the OBESITY SISTERS. Even though they come from the same parent (the adipose cell), they act differently from each other. Most important, they need a different nutritional approach.

Let's see how each affects our body and how I have treated them:

MALNUTRITION/UNDERNUTRITION: Malnutrition/undernutrition will make you gain fat in the abdomen. It is called abdominal fat.

If you have read or heard anything about excess body fat, and I hope you have, you know that this is the most dangerous one because it increases the risk of getting diabetes, high blood pressure, heart disease, stroke, high cholesterol, dementia, and cancer.

And it turns out that you can accumulate abdominal fat even when you are eating a balanced meal!

Here is an example: when a woman is poorly nourished while pregnant, she programs her child to accumulate abdominal fat at around age 30. What a bad deal: to gain waistline without having any say in the matter!

And children from ages 5 to 9 who eat less than what they should increase their risk of developing excess body fat in their teens.

Adults don't escape either since whatever they lose on a strict diet will be recovered mainly on their waist! What a crummy deal: to end with more unhealthy fat after trying your best to lose it!

How do you get rid of abdominal fat?

You do it with a balanced meal plan of no less than 1,300 calories, and this is what you will find in this book!

How long do you have to wait to see results? It all depends on how much and how long you've been malnourished. The longer you've had a bulging belly, the more you will have to wait to see your waistline trim down.

OVERNUTRITION: This fat accumulates mainly on gluteus, hips, thighs, arms, and breasts. It is called gluteal fat.

Gluteal fat is different from abdominal fat, and fortunately, it is not related to increased chances of getting hit with some disease.

Gluteal fat has an extraordinary work to do in women since it is utilized for breastfeeding. Mother's milk has over 50% of fat that comes precisely from fat on her hips!

Gluteal fat has been humanity's silo for thousands and thousands of years. If it were not for gluteal fat, I would not be writing this book, and you would not be reading it, i.e. humanity would have disappeared from the face of the earth. You see, when a woman breastfeeds, she can sustain a child even with minimal food supply if she has gluteal fat.

How do you get rid of this type of fat?

It cannot be with under-nutrition/malnutrition since the body will protect this fat just in case it must be used for breastfeeding, and it cannot be with diets low in carbs and high in fats, or even with a diet with 30% fat.

You must first turn off Starvation Mode with a balanced meal (at least 1,300 calories per day) and then shift the balance to 27% fats. Since reducing fats doesn't work, you increase good carbs. The easy way to do this is to apply this book's recommendations for at least three weeks, and then increase fruits, rice, cornbread, and pasta gradually to your meal plan until you start to see gluteal fat go away.

PROLONGED AND FREQUENT FASTING: This fat accumulates under the skin, which is why it is called subcutaneous fat.

The best place to identify this fat is measuring the chest at the lowest part of the sternum. Women hate this fat because it splurges under and over their bras. This fat is entirely differently from abdominal (visceral) and gluteal fat. It has different receptors and is related to a substance called lipoprotein lipase, which is liberated from the body when there is prolonged fasting.

How do you eliminate this type of body fat?

It would seem to be the easiest fat to remove since all you must do is to stop fasting. It means that you must eat every two to four hours and preferably establish specific times for breakfast, lunch, and dinner.

For years, I played with diets where people ate every hour, and I discovered that thoracic fat went down NO MATTER WHAT I GAVE THEM if they did it every hour. It means that you can lose subcutaneous fat even with apple pies, potato chips, or whatever you fancy! Yum-yum!

But, and here is the catch, having something every hour is hard to do. First, it's not normal for our body to receive food every hour, so you end up forcing yourself to eat even when not hungry. And second, it's not easy to stop your daily activities to find something to eat every hour. But then again, all you must do to lose thoracic fat is eat frequently!

STRESS: This fat accumulates in the lower abdomen. I call it stress fat.

There is a huge collage of causing factors since you can get fat from stress at work, from not sleeping your seven or eight hours (for whatever reason), from infections like Chickenpox, Adenovirus, and Firmicutes, from thoracic and abdominal surgeries like hysterectomy or appendectomy, from a tonsillectomy, etc.

How do you eliminate this bulge?

You must treat it with a balanced diet since it is, in fact, abdominal fat, but with a twist, which is using soluble fiber and resistant starch. Weeks 1 and 2 address this fat, and I will explain treatment later.

LOW CALORIC INTAKE: This fat accumulates in the upper part of the chest, creating a thick neck and broad shoulders. I call it shoulders fat.

There is a disease with high cortisol that causes fat buildup in the upper chest. It can also appear when people take cortisone pills for whatever reason. This fat is sometimes called buffalo hump. There is no real under-nutrition or malnutrition, but the person is eating less than what he needs. A balanced 1,600-calorie diet will protect you from abdominal fat, but if you require 2,500 calories or more, you accumulate fat around the upper chest and shoulders.

How do you eliminate this type of body fat?

You must eat over 2,000 balanced calories per day. It is the usual amount that I give to people over 60 years of age, and they obtain quite spectacular results! But you do have to be careful that you're not jumping from Starvation Mode to a 2,000-calorie diet. It could make you gain weight before you start to lose shoulders fat. My advice is to start low and build up your calories gradually.

NEO-FORMATIONS: This fat accumulates wherever she wants to, ignoring all the other sisters! Therefore, I call them neo-formations.

Some places are common grounds for this lady, such as pouches in front of armpits, love handles, the bags that form between the thighs right under the genitals, fat around the belly button, and any place she fancies. She acts independently of all the other causes, and she can appear even in thin people.

How do you eliminate this type of body fat?

You must eat high quantities of green-leafy vegetables. The ones that work the best are called power greens, and both mustard greens and watercress excel in helping you get rid of these bumps. But other greens also work, including kale, collard greens, bok choi, and chard. You can either cook them or juice them. I do not recommend blending these greens because quantities needed are so large that they will usually cause bloating. You also must be careful of mixing up your greens and spreading them out during the week, because high consumption of kale and bok choi may cause hypothyroidism. Again, this strategy will not work if you are in Starvation Mode.

Why do some people have all these sisters?

You can be eating fewer legumes, fruits and vegetables than you should (waistline), be overeating fats (hips), skipping meals (chest), eating fewer calories than what you should (shoulders), not enough greens (neo-formations) and have chronic uncontrolled stress (lower abdomen). Oh, and neo-formations can appear in ANYONE AND ANYWHERE.

Here is another point to consider: accumulation of excess body fat can be an ongoing event, or it can be evidence of past inappropriate eating habits:

If your thighs have been getting thicker lately, you are currently eating more fat than you can burn. If thighs got big years ago, but they are currently the same, you over-ate at some point in your life, but you are not doing it anymore. It holds true for abdominal fat, gluteal fat, subcutaneous fat, stress fat, shoulders fat, and neo-formations. I call these stable fat stores the Fat Scars of inappropriate eating habits.

So, which poor eating habit do you have? Where do you have excess fat?

Disappointed?

You should be if you tried to get rid of your excess body fat with only one type of diet, i.e. Atkins, Sears, Scarsdale, Weight Watchers, etc., etc., etc.

Since each body fat has a different trigger, each one needs special attention. One diet will not reduce fat from all your body.

As a matter of fact, the fat that you almost always lose, the easiest one of all, is subcutaneous fat, not because of your diet, but because nearly every diet asks you to eat at least three meals per day.

Most diets will also encourage you to increase green leafy vegetables, and this might help you lose some abdominal fat and neo-formations, but it's not going to be that much:

With traditional low-calorie diets, people lose a little less than two inches (5 cm) of waistline in six months. My patients lose more than two inches ON THE

AVERAGE after four weeks. There is no way to compare what you get with this book to the other crummy diets.

Recapitulating: in the treatment of all these sisters, there is a common path that begins with at least 1,300 calories of a balanced meal spread out in many intakes. Once you have covered this base, you can start working on specific parts of your body that bother you the most.

No one ever said that it was easy, but you can do it.

All you need is discipline and patience.

And most important, you cannot target fat loss in specific parts of your body until you have had enough balanced foods to override Starvation Mode.

Now, it might be that what you have just read is hard to digest, and that is fine. No worries. At least now you know that what you have always been doing will NEVER help you obtain long-term results.

So, just how do you lose the fat never to regain it again?

Let's find out!

HOW CAN WE AVOID EXCESS BODY FAT?

After years of researching, working on different theories, and failing with all my efforts to help people permanently lose excess fat, I finally discovered the simple tool that Mother Nature uses to keep naturally thin people thin: FOOD. To understand this, we must focus our attention on naturally thin people instead of people with excess body fat.

We all have naturally thin friends who eat anything they want and do it all day long. They violate all dieting rules and still maintain a thin body.

They also shatter all theories about why you get excess body fat. For example:

•Carbs are fattening.

•Fats make you fat.

•Everything makes you fat.

Just how do naturally thin people maintain their svelte figures even when eating whatever they want? The answer is quite simple: by eating in abundance and with balance. They aren't aware of what they're doing, or how they do it, and most important, they don't even care!

The following explanation uses terminologies that may be confusing to laypeople, and even more so if you're not a math whiz. But don't worry if you get lost. Excess body fat can only be eliminated through discipline and patience anyway. Thousands of patients are now naturally thin without understanding why, and on the other side, many people understand everything and remain fat because they don't change the way they eat.

Various international health organizations, starting with the WHO, have published that we should eat a diet with 55% carbohydrates, 15% proteins, and 30% fats. A nutrition program that reflects these proportions is called a balanced meal or program.

Fortunately, these percentages have margins, which makes it easier to eat a balanced meal. Carbohydrates can range from 50% to 60%, fats from 25% to 35% and proteins from 13% to 20% (a far narrower range).

You must also include at least 25 grams of fiber in your diet.

Besides eating in balance, you should eat at least three times per day. It is also important to eat enough calories: at least 1500 calories per day.

If you cover these requirements – balance, frequency, and sufficiency – the body stays thin. But if you stray from these numbers with bad choices (eating out of balance, infrequently or insufficiently) your body defends itself by storing fat through Starvation Mode. Malnutrition (and Starvation Mode) generates excess body fat sooner or later.

You become fat when you don't eat right and when you don't eat enough of the right things.

The most destructive way of trying to eliminate excess body fat is through strict diets because they trigger even more Starvation Mode. Therefore, you regain weight and gain even more when you stop a diet.

After two years, people on strict diets weigh 120% of what they did when they started. They end weighing 20% more!

Instead of starving yourself, even more, eat enough of a balanced diet to reverse Starvation Mode. Once you change Starvation Mode, you will naturally lose excess body fat. But it will require patience, a trait that is minimal or absent in almost anyone who starts a weight loss diet.

Some might even gain weight and volume when going on a healthy, balanced and sufficient diet. Why?

It is due to severe undernutrition that is being corrected by our bodies. You do run the risk of gaining some weight and inches with a balanced and abundant diet. Those with severe Starvation Mode will pack some excess body fat at first. But keep in mind that according to statistics you end up with 20% more weight if you use a traditional low-calorie diet anyway. Don't you think that it's way better to gain a little at first, and be thin two years later?

One way out of this slight dilemma is to start with small portions of balanced foods and increase your portions slowly. It is the approach of this book.

If you're feeling bold, you can start out with abundance (Week 4 on out), but if you're terrified of weight gain, start with Week 1, and gradually add more food and food groups as you go along.

Now, let's say that for some non-logical reason you ate as little as possible on Week 1 and gained weight anyway: this means you have severe malnutrition and must see a nutritionist who will help you recover from it.

What about eating too many carbs, proteins, and fats?

Currently, many scientists now agree that proteins, slowly absorbing carbohydrates and raw vegetable fats will unlikely and by themselves cause accumulation of excess body fat.

First, our body has self-regulating mechanisms that stop us from overeating these foods. And even if we do overeat, we have a fabulous response called Thermogenesis that burns off those excess calories. Thermogenesis is active if we do not have Starvation Mode.

To date, the only food that has been shown to quickly generates excess body fat when eaten in excess is certain types of fat.

There are different types of fats: saturated (butter, cream, lard, etc.), polyunsaturated (fats found in corn, safflower and sunflower oils, etc.), and monounsaturated (olive, canola, and avocado oils). The ones that could generate excess body fat are saturated fats obtained from land-based animals and heated vegetable fats.

The current recommendation is to reduce your intake of saturated fats by increasing mono or polyunsaturated fats. Saturated fats cannot be eliminated from the diet because that breaks nutritional balance, triggers Starvation Mode, and therefore, makes your body accumulate excess body fat.

It is a game of percentages: too little and too much will make you fat! So, what percentage of fats can we eat for a safe loss of fat?

In my practice, I have found that menus with 27% to 33% fat achieve what I call "stable fat loss," i.e. it's hard for you to regain what you lost even when you stop eating a balanced diet and eat disastrously for a couple of weeks.

Taking this one step further, I created diets with an exact 30% fat content, and the most extraordinary changes happened. People lost more waistline than from any other part of the body!

This formula is the basis for my book Diets Make You Fat – Eating Makes You Thin, and I also applied it to my Changing Your Eating Habits Workshop. It is the primary distribution I recommend in this book and my daily work. Why?

A bulging waistline increases the risk of developing diabetes, heart disease, stroke, cancer and reduced testosterone. That is why you must first eliminate intra-abdominal fat.

When I reduced dietary fat to 27%, volume was reduced preferably around the hips, thighs, and arms. As you can imagine, it delighted my female patients with bulging hips.

When I increased my patients' protein intake to 20%, emphasizing good quality protein, I discovered that people would lose volume from upper abdomen and cheeks. When I used vegetable based protein instead, the flabby skin caused by the previous dieting tightened up. Isn't that fabulous?

I recently discovered a way to reduce abdominal fat that accumulates between your belly button and pubic bone. How this is done is explained in Week 1.

GETTING BETTER RESULTS

The idea of eating more to lose excess body fat has been around for dozens of years. I would dare say that every single new diet book that has been published for the past ten years begins with this idea.

The scientific name for these of diets is AD LIBITUM. Make a search on the Internet for this word and you will obtain millions of hits.

Then, why is it that eating to become thin has not become wildly popular?

This is because people make a huge number of mistakes when applying this, and by the way, any other diet plan.

These mistakes have nothing to do with discipline, motivation, or resolve.

The error lies in **faulty thought processes**, and if you do not understand and change them, you will be unsuccessful in eradicating your excess body fat.

You have an excellent shot at getting rid of excess body fat forever, and at the same time obtaining the body of your dreams! Oh, and your doctor will also congratulate you for your blood work and your healthy bones!

So, go for it and follow the rules of the game just the way they're laid out. Please avoid being creative and original.

If you do not follow these simple rules, you just might lose massive amounts of weight and volume, but you will be fueling the risk of packing on excess pounds again, and you don't want or need that, do you?

Perhaps when people hear "eat to lose it" for the first time, they consider it to be total madness or a magical solution, or worse still, something that will happen spontaneously. The sad news is that it doesn't.

On the other hand, it isn't magic. You can't use a magic wand with only the desire to make it work. You need commitment and discipline.

So, let me share with you some of the most common **faulty thought processes** which put unsurmountable stumbling blocks in your way. Avoid them, and you just might obtain spectacular results!

Lack of objective evidence: This is the worst faulty thought process of all. You see, you WILL NOT FEEL anything when on this program, and therefore you will leave it thinking that it is not working.

I strongly urge you to **use objective evidence** to establish what is going on with your body. Weigh yourself, measure your body, take before and after photos and videos, try on non-elastic clothing that did not fit anymore.

Do not pay attention to what you FEEL, because what you feel is almost always not what is really happening. By the way, we use this faulty thought process in almost every area of our life. We have not been taught to challenge what we feel with objective evidence.

If we go around life making decisions based on what we feel, we will be creating a disastrous lifestyle. We all have the right to feel how we want to feel, but when it comes to deciding what to do with these feelings, we had better obtain **objective evidence** to make the right decisions.

So, do not trust yourself about what you feel, and above all, do not make decisions based only on those feelings.

Fear of food: This is faulty thought process number two. When people make decisions based solely on fear, they will almost always obtain disastrous results. Do not allow yourself to make nutritional choices based on fear.

If you're like most dieters, you've tried a whole range of programs that are, frankly, ridiculous, like eliminating something because "it makes you fat". If you think this is probably just one more ridiculous strategy, you have nothing to lose by trying it – after all, you've already tried other crazy methods! And if it works, you've got proof that it's okay to keep eating despite the fear you may have of food.

Guilt: This is faulty thought process number three. Just ask yourself, how many hours of guilt do you need to lose one pound? The answer is none because guilt does not make you lose weight when you do not follow the program.

Here's where people with obese generating habits experience "ecstasy and agony": ecstasy when they satisfy a craving and agony over having eaten it. They usually try to "cleanse" their guilt by eating less or even by severe fasting. This only increases the probability of splurging AGAIN when famine hits hard enough, even when terrified of food. The vicious cycle closes: fear, binging, guilt, fasting, fear, binging, guilt, fasting, etc.

When eating a little "extra," just go back to eating what the program recommends. Let's say you ended up gorging on a pound of pastries, and you aren't hungry at dinnertime. "Punishment" will be to eat what's for dinner, even when not hungry!

Believe me; this is the most logical and sensible attitude that can help you permanently lose excess fat.

Poor administration: People have the erroneous idea that things will happen magically with just the decision to do them. This is not so.

Poor administration is a severe problem – and a prevalent one today. We have many responsibilities: career, kids, relationships, etc. It can seem as if there is no time to prepare your nutritional program.

The most frequent complaint I hear is that there's no time to prepare meals or even to eat what's already prepared. Pledge to make time to eat what your body requires. Perhaps what you need most is not to start the best diet in the world, but to better administer your hectic schedule.

Perfectionism: This can affect the program negatively in two ways: first, it keeps you from even starting the program if there is any possibility of failure: since it's always possible to make mistakes, the perfectionist never starts. Second, once a perfectionist does start a program and makes a mistake, he drops it. He wants to do things so perfectly that he never gets them done. To err is human, and the best attitude you can have is the following: If you made mistakes yesterday, it doesn't matter … keep on going today anyway, and don't worry about tomorrow until it comes.

Adherence: This is a term used by doctors to refer to how diligently patients apply their treatments. Ideally, they should follow prescribed dosage the recommended number of times and for the length of time indicated. In the United States, researchers have conducted numerous studies on adherence, and they found that patients only follow 80% of doctor's recommendations.

If you want to become naturally thin, follow this program as diligently as possible (but not with a perfectionist attitude). You might fail to follow the program in three ways:

Eating more than what I recommend. It is a minor boo-boo, for as long as you stick to the rest of the program, you will reduce weight and measurements anyway, albeit more slowly.

Eating less than what I recommend: It is a grave error that condemns your body to gain back all you have lost in the long run. Eat recommended quantities of food, even if you sometimes don't have an appetite, and even if you previously have gorged on something that was not in your plan.

Reducing the number of meals: I prescribe seven small meals per day. If you eat fewer meals per day, you will lose fat from your chest more slowly. If you skip a meal for whatever reason, eat it at some other point in the day, even when not hungry.

The best way to establish adherence is to take note of everything you eat. Don't trust memory, because sooner or later you'll be racking your brain trying to remember if you ate pastries or lettuce yesterday.

Write down all that you eat with obsessive perfection. Take photos of every single food that goes inside of you, journal what you eat and even what you think about what you are doing.

One research demonstrated that people could lose up to 35 pounds of excess weight when they journal what they eat! This is more than what is lost with bariatric surgery.

So, if you want to obtain surgical type results, go for it, and start journaling your journey to a naturally thin body!

Conclusions:

Eat the way this book recommends, even if you are a perfectionist, feel fear or guilt, don't believe it will work, don't have the time or any other excuse you might come up with to stop eating.

READY, SET, GO!

How do you turn theory into practice and get rid of body fat the right way? I have created three different approaches:

My book How to Cure Obesity recommends a special eating order: fruits and vegetables first, animal and vegetable protein second, and finally foods with processed sugars and fats. Although it works, we don't usually eat that way. We eat a sandwich, not lettuce and tomatoes first, cheese second, bread third and finally mayonnaise!

My book Diets Make You Fat - Eating Makes You Thin has a mixed meal program that holds you by the hand and gives out exactly what you need to eat every day of the week for seven consecutive weeks. Recommendations were arranged to obtain nutritional balance after eating all foods in a 24-hour period. The advantage is that it is based it on mixed meals, i.e. you eat a typical sandwich. But you must eat exactly how it's laid out, and you have little room for variety or creativity.

In this book, I am presenting a new plan which is balanced and at the same time flexible:

BASIC MEALS AND BALANCED PACKS:

This new strategy offers "Basic Meals" that include the following:

Early Morning Snack
Mid-Morning Snack
Main Meal
Mid-Afternoon Snack
Late Evening Snack

When you have eaten all these five meals, you will have obtained a nutritionally balanced 24-hour program.

There is a total of eight "Basic Meals", starting in week 1 and ending with week 8. What is the difference between them? I increase calories as weeks advance, as well as new food groups.

I did not include breakfast and dinners in the "Basic Meals".

"Balanced Packs" will be used for breakfast and dinner. "Balanced Packs" have by themselves the ingredients for nutritional balance. You will learn how to prepare and switch them in any way you like. It means that one day you can have scrambled eggs, the next oats, and on the third day peanut butter and jelly sandwich! No matter which "Balanced Pack" you use, you will be eating a balanced breakfast and dinner.

I will now go into a little bit of information that I hope Nutritionists will enjoy. It is not necessary for everyone to UNDERSTAND to use the program. Even if the next paragraph is not entirely understood, all you really must do is apply the rules. Here we go:

Each Balanced Pack and each Basic Meal is composed of around 55% carbohydrates, 15% proteins and 30% fats (20% or more of poly or monounsaturated fats and 10% or less of saturated fats). Foods have a low glycemic index during the first weeks. I also included foods with mono and polyunsaturated fatty acids, as well as high in Omega 3 fatty acids.

That was easy, wasn't it? And it gets better:

Toward the end of the book you will be doing something that will be even fun: in Week 8, you will use Special Balanced Packs that are delicious combinations, but which I advise that you eat occasionally (I'll tell you why later).

I have divided the program into three phases, each of which usually causes different types of fat loss:

Strict Phase (Weeks 1, 2 and 3)
Aesthetic Phase (Weeks 4 and 5)
Tasty Phase (Weeks 6, 7 plus Special Basic Meals)

Strict Phase: It causes a rapid loss of weight and measurement. It is structured to whittle down the waist and especially eliminate fat from the lower abdomen (between the belly button and pubic bone).

Aesthetic phase: It slowly reduces excess fat wherever there is any and encourages the body to recover healthy fat where there should be some. A woman's body has a healthy fat accumulation in breasts and hips. Women who diet often lose some of these curves and the aesthetic phase will help them recuperate their beautiful curves.

When you also recover normal fat (also called structural fat) on your face, you will reduce your wrinkles, and you will look ten to twenty years younger.

This phase helps women get a figure that is curvy yet svelte. Muscle mass is usually recovered toning and shaping glutes and calves. Men notice that their legs and arms become more muscular and toned.

Tasty Phase: The body is still experiencing an aesthetic response (losing fat where you should and at the same time recovering fat where you should), but it's much slower because you will add combinations that are not so rigid, but oh so delicious!

Even though fat mobilization slows down, you gain flexibility and variety. And with more flexibility, you are likelier to stick with the program.

Repetition forms a habit, and habits tend to be permanent.

The first few weeks are a bit monotonous because you must repeat a Basic Meal along with the respective Balanced Pack. But don't worry, you will be adding more and more options as the weeks advance.

Once you have completed all the book's recommendations, you are invited to create your meal plans.

Perhaps you may choose to use Basic Meal 4 one day, and switch to Basic Meal 5 the next. There is no right or wrong way to combine meal plans; there's only YOUR WAY!

Once you have mastered this book, it is quite difficult for you to regain lost fat, thus becoming truly naturally thin!

You will also find a special treat at the end of this book.

It has a section that outlines mathematical equations used for loss of fat in specific areas of the body.

There will be two phases in the new era of nutrition:

The first will be to dominate excess body fat. And with the help of this book, I am hoping to help millions and millions of people to become naturally thin!

The second one will be to reshape the body by either reducing or increasing body fat through targeted actions. And wow is this going to be fun!

The equations at the end of the book are meant for dietitians and nutritionists, although those who are very savvy on nutrition software will be able to create their own personalized targeted fat loss programs.

If you are not a nutrition software expert, I have created and uploaded very basic targeted fat loss diets to my Web page boliodiets.

They can help you shape your body the way you want.

There is a monetary cost, a tiny one.

And I do hope that you obtain the same result that thousands of people are already getting. You can see some before and after pictures on my Facebook page Dr. Bolio

WEEK 1

Basic Meal 1

Balanced Pack 1

Balanced Smoothies 1 - 3

Basic Meal 1

Early morning: 1 cup of melon, or cantaloupe, or papaya, or watermelon, or strawberries, or jicama
2 whole raw almonds or 1 whole raw walnut or pecan

Breakfast: Balanced Pack 1: (explained below)

Mid-morning: 1 cup of melon, or cantaloupe, or papaya, or watermelon, or strawberries, or jicama
2 whole raw almonds or 1 whole raw walnut or pecan

Lunch: 2 ounces of tuna canned in water, or turkey breast, or chicken breast (grass-fed or organic)
½ of a medium Haas avocado (80 g of pulp)
2 cups of mixed greens salad
Tea, or coffee (no sugar), as much as you want

Mid-afternoon: 1 cup of melon, or cantaloupe, or papaya, or watermelon, or strawberries, or jicama
2 whole raw almonds or 1 whole raw walnut or pecan

Dinner: Balanced Pack 1 (same as in breakfast)

Late Evening: 1 cup of melon, or cantaloupe, or papaya, or watermelon, or strawberries, or jicama
2 whole raw almonds or 1 whole raw walnut or pecan

AT LEAST 8 GLASSES OF WATER THROUGHOUT THE DAY

Calories	Carbohydrates	Total protein	Total Fat	Saturated Fat	Fiber
449	51%	20%	29%	4%	18g

Note: the calories of this table ONLY correspond to Basic Meal 1. To know the calories for the whole day, add Balanced Pack 1 calories.

Early-morning: It is important that you eat your fruit and raw nuts as soon as you wake up and no more than half an hour after doing so, before your morning shower, workout, and even before getting dressed. Eventually, you will get to the point where your appetite will be the alarm clock. Use an 8-ounce measuring cup to ensure that you have the exact amount.

Now if you have breakfast as soon as you wake up, please continue with this excellent habit. Just have your fruit with seeds together with your breakfast.

Breakfast: Add Balanced Pack 1 as described in detail below. Ideally, you should have your breakfast no later than 2 hours after waking up.

Mid-morning: Eat your specified fruit with raw almonds or walnut 2 to 3 hours after breakfast, and wait for 2 to 3 more hours before having lunch.

Lunch: Weigh your protein after cooking. If you have cellulite or are in a hurry to lose weight, your best option is fish. A word of caution with large cold-water fish: due to mercury content, the USDA recommends that we eat no more than 12 ounces per week of tuna or salmon. You can eat free amounts of smaller fish such as herring, mackerel, and sardines.

Weigh your 80 g (2.6 ounces) of Hass avocados without skin and seed.

You can use any green vegetables for your salads, such as lettuce, spinach, celery, arugula, broccoli, etc. You can also add small quantities of carrots, corn, and tubers like potatoes, yams, etc. to give it more flavor

It is entirely possible that this lunch will not leave you satiated (full) and to solve this; you have two options: the best one is to increase vegetables since you can eat as many as you want at any moment of the day. The other one is to add one of the tostadas recommended for breakfast and dinner.

Drink at least eight cups of plain water each day (even more in hot weather), and learn to enjoy it as it is. If you desire flavor enhancement, you may add coffee, a bit of hibiscus tea, lemon juice, green or black tea, cucumber slices, mint leaves, orange peels, etc.

When seasoning, use condiments that have been reported to generate fat loss: coffee, green or black tea, mate tea, mustard seeds, Himalayan salt, pepper, lemon juice, miso powder, spicy salsa or sauce, apple cider vinegar, ginger, curcumin, garlic, onions and Paradise grains. Mustard seeds and Paradise Grains may increase metabolism by 25%. Wow!

If you prepare food with great seasonings, no one in your family will know you haven't cooked with oil. It is an excellent move, as I will explain later.

Mid-afternoon: Eat any recommended fruit together with raw nuts or almonds 2 to 3 hours after eating lunch. It will work perfectly for those who already snack between 2 and 3 PM. If you have your dinner 8 hours or more after lunch, you can add an extra serving of fruit with seeds. For example, lunch at 12, one fruit snack at 3, another fruit snack at 6, and dinner at 9.

Dinner: Balanced Pack 1 as described below.

Late evening: Some people sleep immediately after going to bed. Others watch TV, read, and/or chat with family members before going to sleep. Your last snack should be after these activities and right before brushing your teeth to go to sleep.

Be very diligent in drinking eight or more glasses of water. This week is very high in fiber, and you do not want to get abdominal cramps from lack of water. Recent research has reported that drinking two glasses of water before a meal slightly increases your metabolism. Therefore, it would be a very good idea to drink two glasses before breakfast, lunch, and dinner, and two more glasses at any other moment of the day.

I have tried to account for the general population's most common eating habits. If this schedule doesn't fit your daily routine (for example if you work at night), you can move meals around to fit you, since the order of intake does not affect how quickly you lose weight or volume. Just program your day to eat something every 2 to 3 hours if you're awake.

Balanced Pack 1

For breakfast and dinner

1 toasted (oven roasted) corn tortilla or ¼ cup cooked corn (serve cold)
¼ of a medium-sized avocado (40 g of pulp)
¼ cup of cooked mashed beans
½ cup of cooked or raw vegetables
1 ounce of low-fat cheese
2 ounces of fruit juice (any type without any added sugar)

Calories	Carbohydrates	T. protein	Total Fat	Saturated Fat	Fiber
248	56%	16%	28%	8%	9 grams

The combination of toasted corn tortilla (also called tostada) with avocado, beans, cheese, fruit juice, and vegetables is a fabulous one that promotes:

Rapid loss of body measurements

Reduction of bad cholesterol and high triglycerides in the blood

Cellulite reduction

Loss of lower abdominal fat

Out of all the Balanced Packs in this book, Balanced Pack 1 is the most powerful one. It has the unique ability to reduce fat in a challenging area of the body, the lower abdomen.

Lars Sjörström reported in Obesity Theory and Therapy (1996) that lower abdominal fat is associated with an increase of fat in the retroperitoneum (behind the small intestine), and is related to many health hazards. Retro-peritoneal fat can increase bad cholesterol and triglycerides as well as the risk of heart attacks and stroke. And most important for all dieters, it can ruin the best weight loss programs.

I discovered years ago that when lower abdomen circumference was the same or greater than breast or hips, there would be minimal or null results from any weight loss program. I coined this phenomenon Metabolic Lockdown.

Three factors combine to generate an accumulation of lower abdominal fat and Metabolic Lockdown:

1. Multiple and severe incidents of malnutrition (severe dieting, major surgery, tonsillectomy, debilitating diseases, etc.).

2. A family history of diabetes, high blood pressure and/or hyperlipidemia.

3. Chronic persistent stress.

None of these three elements cause Metabolic Lockdown by themselves, although every single one does make you lose weight and inches at a slower rate. But oh, do they cause problems when two or more get together!

Major surgeries such as a cesarean section are in a class of their own. Not only can they generate weight gain in the lower abdomen; they can make it almost impossible to lose excess weight with traditional low-calorie diets. These people must use an entirely different nutritional program outside of the scope of this book. You can get that program at my Web page boliodiets.

For years, it was impossible for me to help patients in Metabolic Lockdown. Every program would fail, including absolute fasting, very low-calorie diets, low-carb or no-carb diets, low-fat diets, rotation diets, etc.

If they lost weight, abdominal measurements did not change or decreased with exasperating slowness and worse still, breast, glutes, and calves were lost instead of visceral fat. Reread it: if they lost weight, it was because they were losing muscle, bone mass, and normal or structural fat. And let me tell you that this is the WORST thing that can happen with any weight loss program.

So, you can imagine how thrilled I was when I created this fabulous combination of tostadas, beans, low-fat cheese, avocado, and veggies that open the Metabolic Lockdown and blast lower abdominal fat!

If you have Metabolic Lockdown, you will finally be able to lose excess body fat, but you will still lose it slower than everyone else.

Balanced Pack 1 is the most powerful one for targeting lower abdominal fat, and getting rid of that paunch is the biggest priority for whoever has it. It is also important for health reasons since those with diabetes, cholesterol, and high blood pressure will almost always gain better control these ailments when the lower abdomen is reduced.

So, when should you eat this awesome fat-blasting Balanced Pack?

You will consume it at breakfast and dinner, and you can even use it any time of the day that you feel like it if you prepare it the same way.

Just keep in mind that it is always better to increase your caloric intake in the morning instead of later in the day. If you are going to add tostadas, try doing it before 2 pm.

If you do not have access to corn tortillas, switch out the toasted tortilla for 1/3 cup of cooked corn, either white or yellow, but in my case, I enjoy tostadas way more than cooked corn. Ok, I do like corn, but I must spice it up with sea salt, lemon juice, some vinegar and lots of hot sauce!

It is EXTREMELY IMPORTANT that you eat either corn or tostadas and beans cold or at least at room temperature. To understand why, read up on resistant starch. I believe resistant starch targets lower abdominal fat.

45

I will repeat it again: eat all tostada ingredients COLD! Now I want you to read this paragraph once more and take this instruction to heart.

Avoid commercially made, pre-packaged tostadas that are fried in oil. You can buy packaged oven baked corn tortillas with less than 1 gram of fat per serving at Latino supermarkets.

You can also toast your soft corn tortillas: use a wire grill basket over the burner of your stove, holding it high enough over the flame to avoid burning it. You can also bake it, lay it over the electric stove, or even pop it in the microwave if you do not fry it. Leave it crunchy but not black.

Do not reheat your tostadas: eat them at room temperature (have I mention that before?).

MAGICAL AVOCADOES

Avocados are a wonder fruit! I consider it to be the best food on the planet. Therefore, I chose it as the core food for obtaining healthy fats. Remember that a balanced diet has around 30% of fat, and there is no better way to eat them than through avocados.

Below is a partial list of the many benefits of avocado:

Improves digestion, reduces bad breath by killing bacteria, helps obtain younger and supple skin, protects the liver through beta-carotene and lycopene, protects the eyes through zeaxanthin, reduces cholesterol through beta-sitosterol, reduces blood pressure through high potassium content, contains 40% of daily vitamin K requirements, reduces morning sickness in pregnancy, reduces arthritis, has anti-cancer properties, is an excellent anti-oxidant, reduces age-related memory loss, is anti-aging, makes you lose weight, makes you lose abdominal fat, slows down the aging process through xanthophyll, increases the absorption of other heathy nutrients, and contains a sugar that helps control glucose metabolism.

You can switch out your ¼ avocado for a teaspoon of olive oil or coconut oil, but I highly advise against it because you will be losing all the benefits obtained from this wonder fruit.

Use preferably black beans, although you can switch them out for other types of beans to avoid boredom. Cook and mash your beans without adding oil. Add any spice that you wish to season them. You can also buy refried beans if they contain less than 1 gram of fat per serving. Let your beans cool down and spread them cold over your tostadas.

With regards to the veggies, pick anything you like, including tubers such as sweet potatoes. Potatoes also contain resistant starch, which can increase your ability to burn fat, but remember to eat them cold after cooking.

Because tostadas will be repeated for breakfast and dinner for a whole week, vary the veggies that go on top so that you don't get bored of this meal. One day you can use mushrooms, on another red tomatoes and lettuce, and on a third day, cooked or raw spinach.

You should also use condiments like pepper, cumin, aromatic herbs, soy sauce, Worcestershire sauce, etc. Remember to include condiments that have been reported to generate fat loss: Himalayan salt, ginger, curcumin, pepper, lemon juice, miso powder, spicy salsa or sauce, apple cider vinegar, garlic, onions, coffee, green or black tea, mate tea, mustard and Paradise grains. Mustard and Paradise grains increase metabolism by 25%.

Low-fat cheese should have between 5 and 6 grams of fat per ounce of serving. If it isn't this amount, don't worry if the package says low fat or made from part skim milk.

Fruit juice can be homemade, or store bought. If you buy it at a market, it should ideally be organic. Both cherry juice and grapefruit juice have been reported to assist with fat loss, but do not overuse them, and above all, tell your doctor if you plan on using grapefruit juice in your menu.

The beauty of Balanced Pack 1 is that you can repeat it as many times as needed per day, whenever needed, and you'll still lose weight and measurements! If you are hungry at breakfast one morning, add one, two, three or four more tostadas (with all the ingredients). You'll still be fine. You can also use them as a snack between meals.

For the magic to work, it is critical to use the exact ingredients, in recommended portions. It's something like preparing multiple batches of a recipe you like – for the recipe to come out right every time, you must add the same ingredients in the same quantities.

If you decide to eat another tostada, you must add another ¼ cup of boiled beans, another ¼ of an avocado, another ounce of low-fat cheese, another ½ cup of vegetables, and another 2 ounces of fruit juice.

If you feel particularly hungry at lunch, you can add one or two more tostadas or as many as needed till you feel full.

Women usually opt for one or two extra tostadas during the day (1,193 to 1,441 calories including Basic Meal 1). Men are typically happy with two to four added tostadas (1,441 to 1,937 calories, including Basic Meal 1).

This will help you to lose weight without going hungry. Always keep in mind that diets which keep you hungry may generate Starvation Mode which will make you regain whatever you've lost, and possibly even more.

The more tostadas you eat, the slower your body measurements might go down, but it will also be transforming you into a naturally thin person.

Apply Basic Meal 1 plus Balanced Pack 1 for seven consecutive days. It is a bit monotonous but straightforward to get the hang of. Over the weeks that follow, I will explain how to put more variety into your diet and continue the road to becoming naturally thin.

What problems might arise when eating this pack?

It is uncommon to experience discomfort, but if it does appear, it could be caused by the following situations:

Bad previous eating habits: If you eat very little fiber, beans can cause a lot of digestive discomforts. Symptoms should disappear by the third week the program. If the discomfort is minimal, you don't have to do anything. But if you are experiencing moderate bloating or even a little pain, you can switch the tostadas for oatmeal. (you will use oatmeal in Balanced Pack 2, and I'll describe ingredients on Week 2.) You can also add pills that help digest beans, and you can get these pills at your preferred pharmacy.

Not chewing your food: some people gulp their food instead of eating it slowly. When you do take your time to eat, you are making it easier on your stomach to finish digesting food and getting it ready for absorption. Saliva is also essential for digestion, especially for carbohydrates. Get into the habit of totally chewing at least your Balanced Pack 1.

Irritable bowel: This is frequently associated with stress, but can also happen when physical activity is minimal. If you have Irritable Bowel Syndrome, consider the possibility of applying the Induction Diet that you can buy at my Web page boliodiets.

You might also have to check with your doctor possible treatments to eliminate discomfort.

Parasites and/or fungus: Some parasites, especially amoebas and giardia, can cause digestive disturbances that become even more intense with carbohydrates, and this is called sugar intolerance. Another critter that can cause sugar intolerance is an overgrowth of Candida Albicans.

You might need to follow specific medical treatment to stop digestive discomfort caused by these parasites and fungi.

Dysbiosis: this is an improper balance of gut bacteria, where there is an overgrowth of species that generate inflammation with severe bloating and even diarrhea. This event requires two special diets: Gut Healing Diet and Probiotics Diet, which you can download at my Web page boliodiets.

I also highly recommend a diet prescribed by Dr. Gerard E. Mullin in his book The Gut Balance Revolution. After you follow any of these diets, you should be able to do this book without symptoms.

Weight gain and expanded body measurements: This is not common, but when it does occur, don't worry. Very low-calorie diets and low carb diets make you gain weight when you stop them abruptly.

If you are currently on a very low-cal, or a low-carb diet, you can do two things before starting this diet to reduce the possibility of gaining weight:

One is to eat whatever your heart desires for two or three days before beginning the plan. A lot of people have "going away parties" before starting a diet, and it's not a bad idea. Yeah, you might gain some weight, but so what? It's always so much easier to start a diet on a full stomach, and the weight you gain is going to disappear anyway!

The other option is a lot stricter, and this is to do partial fasting for two days where you only eat fruit every two hours. You can eat as much as you want of any fruit. This is a great option for people who are on low carb diets.

There is a third option: you can download the Induction Diet at my Web page boliodiets. This diet helps you stabilize your weight when leaving most strict diets. After the week of the Induction Diet, you should be able to start this book's plans without any weight gain.

You can use any one of these options if you don't have high or low blood glucose. If you have any of these, stick it out with this book.

The Six O'clock Bulge: abdominal bloating sometimes makes you wrongly conclude that you're getting fat. I call this the "six o'clock bulge," because clothes fit tighter in the evening. The next morning, when clothes fit better, we calm down, to again experience another emotional turmoil at night, believing we've gotten fat again.

To avoid these misunderstandings, put on an article of non-elastic clothing from "before the bulge" (something that used to fit well but that is not comfortable anymore), immediately upon waking up, when there is minimal abdominal bloating. If your clothing starts feeling more comfortable, you are indeed losing excess fat, despite experiencing the "six o'clock bulge."

Over time, when your body begins to digest fiber more efficiently, the "six o'clock bulge" will go away or be reduced. You may notice this around the second or third week of the program.

Menstrual Period: If your menstrual period is regular, you will probably see a lot of changes, since it will stop being regular. It happens with any diet that makes you lose fat. Your period should become normal again when you reach a stable weight.

Women should also keep in mind that the menstrual period increases weight and measurements, especially breasts and lower abdomen. If gaining weight causes your panic attacks, start the program after your period has ended and your weight has gone back to normal.

Traveling: when you travel to hot climates, the weight will go up. It is because of fluid retention and not the accumulation of fat. Alcoholic drinks also cause fluid retention. Suntans and sunburns cause even more fluid retention. All this is temporary and does not mean you are getting fat.

To reduce fluid retention when traveling to hot weather, increase your salt intake two days before traveling. But you can only do this if your doctor has not limited your salt intake. Higher salt intake will usually cause a more stable weight despite abrupt climate changes.

I highly recommend that you apply at least Weeks One to Four of this book before going off on vacations.

PLEASE do not go on a strict diet right before vacations to show off a bikini or cut body at the beach, because you will almost always return from your vacations with more pounds and inches than even before starting the diet.

Strict diets should be applied AFTER you've come back from your vacations. This way you avoid going down and up, and down and up, and down and up, and down and up…

There is a short-cut which may help you reduce symptoms to a minimum and at the same time give you a powerful weapon to adjust this or any other balanced diet to your daily caloric needs:

SMOOTHIES OR MRP
(MEAL REPLACEMENT PLANS)

Try any one of these smoothies which could help you revert Starvation Mode with minimal digestive issues.

Balanced Smoothie 1

For Breakfast and Dinner

4 ounces of plain low-fat yogurt
¼ of a medium-sized avocado (35 grams of pulp)
1 tablespoon of honey (21 grams)

Calories	Carbohydrates	Total protein	Total Fat	Saturated Fat	Fiber
192	55%	15%	30%	8%	2 grams

Since this smoothie is balanced, you can take as many as you wish, but remember that it has lactose. If you are lactose intolerant, you can use lactose-free milk or Lactaid pills.

Hopefully, this smoothie will take care of any symptoms that the tostadas might create, but remember that tostadas revert Metabolic Lockdown.

So as soon as you can, change to your yummy tostadas and enjoy your plan!

Now, try out the next smoothie with kefir (it has none or minimal lactose):

Balanced Smoothie 2

6 ounces of plain low-fat kefir
12 whole almonds or 12 pecan halves
1 medium banana

Calories	Carbohydrates	Total protein	Total Fat	Saturated Fat	Fiber
274	53%	18%	30%	6%	5 grams

Ok, so the calories do go up, but since they are balanced, THEY WILL HELP YOU LOSE EXCESS BODY FAT ANYWAY. Also, consider that kefir has minimal lactose, and if it causes digestive issues, then it is more likely that you have an intolerance to milk protein than to lactose.

For those who have intolerance to lactose and milk protein, I have developed another smoothie that uses powdered vegetable protein

Balanced Smoothie 3

10 grams of vegetable-based protein powder
35 grams of 100% maple syrup
1 teaspoon or 5 grams of olive oil

Calories	Carbohydrates	Total protein	Total Fat	Saturated Fat	Fiber
170	56%	14%	30%	4%	1 grams

This smoothie will be the one that probably causes the least digestive symptoms and the greatest weight loss, but there is a huge problem with it, and it is that it contains ridiculous amounts of vitamins and minerals.

It means that if you are planning on using Balanced Smoothie 3 as your only choice for breakfast and dinner, then you MUST TAKE MULTIVITAMINS. Ask your doctor which ones to use.

If you tolerate all these smoothies, then there is no reason for you not to mix and match, that is, to use all of them during the same day.

You can even repeat smoothies in such a way that you are having one every two hours. For example, a smoothie as soon as you wake up at 6, another smoothie (the higher calorie one) for breakfast at 8, another smoothie at 10 am (probably the maple syrup one), and your regular lunch at 12 pm.

Two or three hours after lunch, you can start drinking a smoothie every two to three hours until your day ends.

These smoothies usually generate spectacular results since you lose weight and inches at a rapid rate if you do not have METABOLIC LOCKDOWN.

Let's suppose you went wild and had a kefir smoothie for breakfast and dinner and added six vegetable protein smoothies during the rest of the day. Why? Because you were hungry and because you can. It will add up to a total of 2017 calorie per day, AND YOU WILL STILL LOSE WEIGHT AND INCHES AT A VERY FAST RATE.

But even if you are obtaining a dramatic loss of weight and volume with only smoothies, you must sooner or later start using the fat-blasting tostadas. Why? Because life is not made up of smoothies and you must LEARN to eat whatever to lose or maintain your weight and volume.

This strategy helped me understand that people can lose weight and inches with a high-calorie balanced diet. I invite nutritionists and doctors to use the same plan: give your patients at least 1,500 balanced calories through shakes and watch how they lose weight and volume! I did the following:

I asked my patients to prepare their shakes and to use them as the base for their diet. The shakes were balanced and most relevant, high in calories.

They could drink at least 1,800 calories in the form of shakes, and afterward, eat whatever they fancied. All of them easily hit over 2,200 calories per day and lost weight as well as inches!

I also learned many interesting things through this approach:

The first one was that people were not afraid of the concept of calories: they were afraid of the visual part of their diet.

They could easily gulp down a 600 calorie shake but would get panic attacks when asked to eat a 200-calorie slice of cheesecake!

It also held true for anorectic and bulimic patients. Even when they knew that they were ingesting a regular or high-calorie diet, they did not have any problem with it if it was through shakes.

But I couldn't ask them to eat regular food because they would not to do it.

Another sad thing that I learned was that people were not willing to leave their shake for a typical balanced meal.

They were not interested in learning to balance their meals with animal protein, vegetables, fruits, cereals, seeds, and grains: they only wanted to gulp down their balanced shakes and lose weight.

I was changing one problem for another one.

And since my objective had always been to obtain a stable loss of excess body fat, I knew for certain that sooner or later my patients would leave their shakes to go back to a disastrous eating pattern, i.e. they would recuperate any lost weight.

So, I am asking you to use these smoothies only during the first days of the program and only in emergency situations, to use all the other balanced packs that this book teaches you, to lose volume slowly, and most important, to learn how to balance out your daily meals!

WEEK 2

Basic Meal 2

Balanced Pack 2

Basic Meal 2

Early morning: **2 ounces of 2% fat milk, or plain low-fat yogurt**
2 crackers (wheat or rice)

Breakfast: Balanced Pack 1 or 2: (read more information below)

Mid-morning: **1 medium apple, banana, grapefruit, or orange**
2 whole raw almonds or 1 whole raw walnut or pecan

Lunch: Fat-free vegetable soup
¼ cup of legumes: black, red, pinto, white, navy, green beans, lentils, or garbanzos (chickpeas)
2 ounces of tuna canned in water, or low-fat cheese, or turkey breast ham or chicken breast (grass-fed or organic)
¼ of a medium Haas avocado (40 g of pulp)
1 cup of mixed greens salad
Tea, or coffee (no sugar), as much as you want

Mid-afternoon: **1 medium apple, banana, grapefruit, or orange**
2 whole raw almonds or 1 whole raw walnut or pecan

Dinner: Balanced Pack 1 or 2 (same as in breakfast)

Late evening: **2 ounces of 2% fat milk, or plain low-fat yogurt**
2 crackers (wheat or rice)

AT LEAST 8 GLASSES OF WATER DURING THE DAY

Calories	Carbohydrates	Total protein	Total Fat	Saturated Fat	Fiber
596	50%	20%	30%	9%	17g

Note: the calories of this table ONLY correspond to Basic Meal 2. To know the calories for the whole day, add calories from Balanced Pack 1 and 2. Food in boldface is added to Basic Meal 2 to increase total caloric intake.

Basic Meal 2 is almost identical to Basic Meal 1, but there are changes that you can spot in bold print. These foods increase calorie from 449 to 596.

This week I made modifications to fruit. On Week 1, I recommend papaya, watermelon, jicama, cantaloupe and honeydew for the morning and noon snacks. Starting in this week, you can use other types of fruit.

A cup of either cantaloupe, honeydew, papaya, pineapple, watermelon, or jicama is considered one fruit serving. Any other fruit (bananas, mangos, etc.) is higher in calories, so for practical purposes, a ½ cup of these types of fruits counts as one serving. A medium-sized apple, pear, banana or mango fill 1 cup and is, therefore, equivalent to 2 servings of fruit.

Bananas, oranges, and apples have a lower satiety index (they fill us up less than papaya, watermelon, cantaloupe, honeydew, or jicama), but they are a lot easier to tote around when you're on the go.

Here are some of the reasons why it is good to add more types of food and eat more calories:

First, because you will still lose weight and inches even when you increase calories over a 24-hour period.

Second, adding more and different foods to the menu gives it more variety and therefore enhances your perception of tastiness, which increases adherence and yields better long-term results.

Third, it gives you the opportunity to re-learn how to eat everything and achieve permanent loss of weight and body measurements.

Fourth, it keeps Starvation Mode from rearing its ugly head again. Any weight loss program that requires minimal caloric intake causes metabolic changes that encourage the body to recover its old weight. When you drastically cut your calories to achieve rapid loss of weight and measurements, it is tantamount to committing nutritional suicide.

Fifth, it encourages an aesthetic loss of volume. You will probably lose weight more slowly, but this may help you obtain a great or even spectacular figure at the end.

99.9% of people who apply this or any other weight loss diet want to do it to look better. There may or may not be a medical reason to lose weight (a spinal injury, joint issues, diabetes, high blood pressure, etc.), but all have a yearning for a more aesthetically attractive body and would like to see quick changes. Heck, even people who DO have a medical need to lose weight will not mind looking better. Who wouldn't?

Unfortunately, a rapid loss of weight or measurements will almost always cause the skin to sag around the face, arms, bust, abdomen, and legs. Also, muscle mass may be lost, especially in glutes and calves, causing you to look ill. Your clothes may fit better, but you will probably look ugly naked.

When your boost your calorie intake, you reduce the risk of losing muscle mass and "regular" or structural fat (i.e. breasts and hips for women, and subcutaneous fat from the face in both sexes). You obtain a slower, but a more aesthetic loss of excess body fat.

Vanity is a potent tool that enables people to apply a rigid, dull, and even dangerous weight loss program. Use your vanity as your ally in this program to lose weight slowly without damaging your health, and you might just be enchanted with the results.

Early Morning: Just as you did during Week 1, eat as soon as you wake up, before showering, working out or even getting dressed. You will get to the point where your appetite will be your alarm clock. Drink low-fat milk with a fat content of 2%, or low-fat flavored yogurt, plus your saltine crackers.

Continue using a measuring cup, or a baby bottle, to obtain the exact portion you need (2 ounces).

You can also switch out the milk or yogurt with 1 cup of cantaloupe, honeydew, papaya, watermelon or strawberries plus six raw almonds or three whole raw walnuts.

Breakfast: Balanced Pack 1 or 2 as explained below.

Mid-morning: Eat your fruit with raw walnuts or almonds 2 to 3 hours after breakfast. Wait for 2 to 3 hours before eating again. If more than 8 hours have passed between breakfast and lunch, eat fruit with walnuts or almonds again in between main meals.

Lunch: Vary your veggies to make your meal tastier. Try soup with onion, tomato puree, broccoli with potatoes, etc. You must prepare your vegetables without oil. You can use any other condiment, such as garlic, salt, pepper, tomato juice, etc. You can also include carrots, peas, etc.

Do not use oil when cooking your beans or lentils. Use any other condiment to season them. Measure your portion with a measuring cup.

During this week, you are still eating a minimal amount of animal protein: 2 ounces of tuna packed in water, or 2 ounces of chicken equivalent to 1 chicken leg, etc. If you have cellulite, prefer the tuna packed in water.

With Haas avocados, weigh your 40 g of pulp without the peel and seed. If you are allergic to avocados (what bad luck!), take a teaspoon of olive, or pure coconut oil, or even eat 1 ounce of olives (15 small olives or 10 large olives).

Learn how to season your foods with fat-free condiments, such as soy sauce or Worcestershire sauce, hot sauce, peppers, salt, lemon or lime juice, etc.

Mid-afternoon: Eat the recommended fruit with the almonds or walnuts 2 to 3 hours after eating lunch. For example, lunch at 12, snack at 3 and dinner at 6. If you eat your dinner more than 8 hours after lunch, add another fruit with seed so that your stomach receives something every two to three hours. For example, lunch at 12, snacks at 3 and 6, and dinner at 9.

Dinner: Balanced Pack 1 or 2.

Before bedtime: Try to eat this last meal right before brushing your teeth and going to sleep. It is to reduces the chance of nighttime hunger.

These recommendations are intended for common dietary habits, so they may not fit your lifestyle. One example is a doctor, nurse, or policeman who works a night shift every other day. If this applies to you, modify meals as needed.

Balanced Pack 2

For breakfast and dinner

½ cup of oats (measured raw)
8 raw almonds or 4 whole raw walnuts or pecans
½ cup of cantaloupe, melon, papaya, watermelon, or strawberries
4 ounces of 2% fat milk
Add water as desired

Calories	Carbohydrates	Total protein	Total Fat	Saturated Fat	Fiber
296	56%	16%	28%	7%	7 grams

Just in case this combination is not filling enough, there is another option that I enjoy more!

Balanced Pack 2A

For breakfast and dinner

½ cup of oats (measured raw)
12 raw almonds or 6 whole raw walnuts or pecans
1 medium apple, banana, or 1 cup of blueberries
8 ounces of 2% fat milk
Add water as desired

Calories	Carbohydrates	Total protein	Total Fat	Saturated Fat	Fiber
445	54%	15%	31%	8%	9 grams

Any of these oatmeal packs encourages the loss of lower belly linked with a buildup of retroperitoneal fat and all sorts of medical issues.

For some people, oatmeal is gross; if this is your story, think of it as choosing between it and your "gross" body. The sensible choice is to eat the oatmeal and lose the excess fat. Improve taste with cinnamon, vanilla extract, or even a little bit of sea salt.

If you still can't stomach oatmeal, here is an alternative; blend all ingredients and have a delicious shake! And if even that grosses you out, just chug it!

Balanced Pack 1 and 2 contain soluble fiber, monounsaturated fats, and low saturated fats. This may help reduce retroperitoneal fat. When you eliminate this fat, it can help you reduce your bad cholesterol.

Lower abdominal fat also increases estrogens in women, which usually causes problems with their period. You will reduce abdominal fat with Balanced Packs 1 and 2, and reduce symptoms during your period, resulting in lighter menstrual flow and less uncomfortable periods.

Women should be cautious with pregnancy issues, because any loss of body fat (through any means, including hunger diets) will reduce estrogen levels, causing a change in the hormonal cycle and usually hastening the onset of menstruation. If you have not gotten pregnant with other diets, be very careful with this one, because proper nutrition increases fertility.

In men, increased abdominal fat reduces testosterone, and when this unhealthy fat disappears, testosterone spikes back up again!

Sex drive grows in both men and women. Singles don't need to fret, for tostadas and oatmeal will not make them sex addicts! But couples on the program will have tons of fun because they look sexier, libido is increased, and for women, the period is a lot easier to deal with. Add increased fertility, and surprise! A visit from the stork may be in the works.

Many women suffering from primary sterility (in other words that would like to get pregnant but can't) have become happy mothers when using this program. If you do not wish a pregnancy now, avoid using the rhythm or condom and use other options that you can discuss with your doctor.

 On Week 2, choose between tostadas and oatmeal at breakfast as well as dinner. Things will start to get interesting!

One day you can choose Balanced Pack 2 or 2A (oatmeal) for both breakfast and dinner, on another day, Balanced Pack 1 (tostadas) for breakfast and dinner, on the third day oatmeal in the morning and tostadas at night.

And remember that if you discover that you are ravenous, decide which of the two Balanced Packs you want to add to your plan. Fascinating, right?

Enjoy your program!

You have very limited options and your plan can feel repetitive by the second week, but just remember that repetition promotes excellence.

We have many repetitive events in our lives that rarely trigger an emotional crisis under normal circumstances. Driving a car, using underwear, taking a bath, and brushing your teeth are all repetitive, monotonous behaviors, but they do not make life annoying and frustrating, o causes an existential crisis.

"Oh, why do I have to brush my teeth again? It is so disheartening that I will feel miserable the rest of the day!" Sounds ridiculous, right?

So, if you do go down that dark path of boredom, I highly recommend you start searching for a mental health professional to help you grow up and be an adult about it.

Oops, maybe I did get a little aggressive, but I have always understood and taught that the worst enemy of someone trying to lose excess body fat is the person himself.

Do not patronize yourself; it's not worth it.

WEEK 3

Basic Meal 3

Balanced Pack 3

Basic Meal 3

Early morning: 2 ounces of 2% fat milk, or plain low-fat yogurt
2 crackers (wheat or rice)

Breakfast: Balanced Pack 1, 2 or 3: (read more information below)

Mid-morning: 1 medium apple, banana, grapefruit, or orange
2 whole raw almonds or 1 whole raw walnut
2 teaspoons of honey

Lunch: Fat-free vegetable soup
¼ cup of legumes: black, red, pinto, white, navy, or green beans, lentils, or garbanzos (chickpeas)
2 ounces of tuna canned in water, low-fat cheese, turkey breast ham, or chicken breast (grass-fed or organic)
¼ of a medium Haas avocado (40 g of pulp)
1 cup of mixed greens salad
Tea, or coffee (no sugar), as much as you want

Mid-afternoon: 1 medium apple, or banana, or grapefruit, or orange
2 whole raw almonds or 1 whole raw walnut or pecan

Dinner: Balanced Pack 1, 2 or 3 (same as in breakfast)

Late evening: 2 ounces of 2% fat milk, or plain low-fat yogurt
2 crackers (wheat or rice)

AT LEAST 8 GLASSES OF WATER THROUGHOUT THE DAY

Calories	Carbohydrates	Total protein	Total Fat	Saturated Fat	Fiber
639	53%	18%	28%	8%	17g

Note: Food in boldface is added in Basic Meal 3 to increase total caloric intake.

Is it okay to use refined sugar like honey when you're trying to slim down?

For years, refined or simple sugars (scientifically referred to as mono- or disaccharides) have been demonized and blamed for everything from addictions to diabetes and early death. To understand the effect of simple sugars on the body, we must first look at the glycemic index, which refers to how quickly the body absorbs carbohydrates.

Our body digests, and therefore absorbs different sugars at varying speeds: mono- and disaccharides are absorbed very quickly, and enter the bloodstream just minutes after we have eaten them. It is the case with agave syrup, glucose, and sucrose (white cane sugar).

Polysaccharides (complex sugars) are absorbed more slowly and take minutes and even hours to reach the bloodstream. It is the case with grapefruit, pears, and sugars contained in ice cream and pasta (spaghetti, macaroni, etc.). It turns out that our body absorbs honey very slowly.

Slowly digested sugars receive a lower number on the glycemic index. For example, grapefruit, which is absorbed slowly, ranks 25 on the glycemic index, while glucose is 138.

Sugars with a low glycemic index cause less insulin liberation. When less insulin is released, this means, in theory, that you reduce the possibility of gaining excess body fat.

The problem with simple sugars is that their rapid absorption makes the body release significant amounts of insulin. Over time, this can cause blood sugar disorders (hypoglycemia, X Syndrome, and Diabetes Mellitus in people with a family history of Diabetes) as well as excess body fat.

Are you lost yet? This area of medicine is somewhat complicated, but we can draw the following simple conclusions from it: the slower sugar is absorbed, the greater the likelihood of slimming down. The more quickly sugar is absorbed, the higher the risk of accumulating fat, as well as elevated triglycerides (fat in the blood) and diabetes.

Considering everything that we have discussed, it would seem unwise to use quickly absorbed sugars in a weight loss diet. However, Dr. John P. Bantle proposed a solution to this dilemma: he reported that eating a simple or refined sugar together with proteins (beef, chicken, etc.) and fats (avocado, etc.) reduced the speed of absorption of that sugar.

Put another way, if you're going to eat refined sugar, white sugar, sugar cubes, jams, jellies, or maple syrup, you should eat it with proteins and fats. Therefore, pastry has a low glycemic index!

So, whenever you eat something sweet between meals, always add raw almonds, nuts, peanuts, or any other seed or nut to provide fat and protein.

That's why Basic Meals 1 and 2 combine fruit with raw almonds as snacks, and Basic Meal 3 adds a little honey to fruit with raw almonds.

This allows you to create tastier slimming diets. You might lose weight more slowly (or you might not), but then again, who's interested in fast weight loss only to gain it all back again, or even more?

If all this still seems complicated, just remember that solution lies in practice, not in theory. I explained food preparation on pages 35 and 45.

Balanced Pack 3

For breakfast and dinner

2 whole medium eggs (organic or cage free)
1 cup of cooked vegetables (red tomatoes, onion, mushrooms peppers, broccoli, etc.)
2 roasted or oven baked corn tortillas (tostadas)
8 ounces of fruit juice

Calories	Carbohydrates	Total protein	Total Fat	Saturated Fat	Fiber
359	53%	17%	30%	8%	6 grams

It is another very popular breakfast, which is very easily balanced.

You can boil your eggs, or scramble them and add whatever veggies you desire. Use cooking spray to keep eggs from sticking to the pan.

Medical organizations used to recommend eating a maximum of 2 whole eggs per week for people over the age of 30. It has changed recently, and now you can eat whole eggs as many times as you want. Just remember that you also want to use your tostadas and your oatmeal to eliminate fat from your lower abdomen (see page 39).

LDL cholesterol, or "bad" cholesterol, has received a lot of attention over the last few years, specifically in its association with heart attacks. Heart attacks are one of the biggest killers in industrialized countries and to reduce their rate, researchers have sought to pinpoint factors that can increase it, and even more important, find out how to change them to decrease the risk.

Various circumstances have been found to increase the possibility of heart attacks: age, gender, smoking, stress, a sedentary lifestyle, Android type excess body fat (accumulation of fat around the waist), in utero malnutrition (in the mother's womb), and high LDL or "bad" cholesterol.

Fortunately, eggs do not seem to increase "bad" cholesterol. On the other hand, they do not reduce it like other foods. These include avocados, beans, oats, omega -3 fatty acids found in cold water fish, and oils from nuts and seeds. Frequent meals also help you reduce bad cholesterol.

This program increases the consumption of fiber, monounsaturated fats and recommends that you eat frequently. Consequently, besides reducing body fat, it may help lower your bad cholesterol.

A study of 100 healthy participants who applied recommendations set out in this book reported a significant reduction of the following lab work: total cholesterol, triglycerides, uric acid, blood glucose, and blood pressure. These changes happened after only two months of treatment.

Occasionally, cholesterol increases during the first few months of treatment. It is usually due to a rise in HDL or "good" cholesterol.

If you have been diagnosed with high cholesterol, triglycerides, blood sugar and/or high blood pressure, this program can help you. But first discuss it with your doctor, who will decide whether to use only this menu, as well as other strategies such as medications, exercise, and stress management.

Now you can eat eggs for breakfast one day, oatmeal another day and tostadas on the third day. And adding eggs will make the diet less monotonous because you can prepare them in so many ways.

I know that the program is still limited and that it may start to feel somewhat dull. But do not despair, for very soon you will have so many options that you might get lost in the jungle of variety.

So, keep your cool, enjoy this week, and get ready for new options.

WEEK 4

Basic Meal 4

Balanced Pack 4

Basic Meal 4

Early morning: 2 ounces of 2% fat milk, or plain low-fat yogurt
2 crackers (wheat or rice)
1-teaspoon honey

Breakfast: Balanced Pack 1, 2, 3 or 4: (read below)

Mid-morning: 1 medium apple, banana, grapefruit, or orange
6 whole raw almonds or 3 whole raw walnuts
2 teaspoons of honey

Lunch: Fat-free vegetable soup
¼ cup of beans: black, red, pinto, white, navy, lentils, or garbanzos (chickpeas)
2 ounces of low-fat animal protein (read below)
½ of a medium Haas avocado (80 g of pulp)
1 cup of mixed greens salad
Water, tea, or coffee (no sugar or milk), as much as you want

Mid-afternoon: 1 medium apple, banana, grapefruit, or orange
4 whole raw almonds or 2 whole raw walnuts
1 teaspoon of honey

Dinner: Balanced Pack 1, 2, 3 or 4 (same as in breakfast)

Late evening: 2 ounces of 2% fat milk, or plain low-fat yogurt
2 crackers (wheat or rice)

AT LEAST 8 GLASSES OF WATER THROUGHOUT THE DAY

Calories	Carbohydrates	Total protein	Total Fat	Saturated Fat	Fiber
795	54%	17%	29%	5%	20g

Note: Food in boldface increases total caloric intake. Basic Meal 4 is like 3, except that it has more honey and seeds. This raises the overall calorie count from 639 to 732 calories.

Animal protein is subdivided into three groups: low, medium and high-fat content.

Wild game is considered low in fat and accumulates 1% total fat, if at all. Other foods like pork rinds have a total fat content of 50%. Fat content can be extremely variable when it comes to animal protein.

Does it make sense to limit animal-derived fats?

Various medical organizations such as the American Diabetes Association, American Cancer Society, American Heart Association, and even the U.S. National Institutes of Health advised limiting animal fats to small quantities.

According to these organizations, diets should contain at most 10% saturated fat from animal protein.

This advice recently changed, and now it turns out that experts are saying, "We were wrong." They have found no clear evidence that animal fat or even total cholesterol from diet affect blood cholesterol. So now it's fine to eat two whole eggs every single day of the week!

When it comes to excess body fat, no matter what type of dietary fat you use, weight and measurements will go down if the total percentage (vegetable and animal) is under 35% - a very generous margin.

You can stay slim eating significant amounts of animal fats – but the cost to your health may be high.

If you eat beef daily, it may increase cholesterol levels in the blood, the rate of arteriosclerosis (hardening of the arteries), and the chance of developing cancer in different parts of the body. It may even trigger premature aging and increase the rate of Alzheimer's.

Some consider that this association does not hold true for organic or grass-fed cattle and that grass-fed, or organic beef will even provide health benefits. It is probably true, but up till now, there have been no long-term population studies that demonstrate a significant beneficial effect. Now if you ask me, I certainly am eating beef, but only grass-fed or organic, and only a couple of times per month.

I do believe that ANY AMOUNT of animal fat may be dangerous to your health if it is not organic or grass fed, not because of the fat, but because fat cells concentrate toxins up to 1,000 times more than other tissues. It is another area of modern day nutrition that I will not cover in this book. I write "modern-day nutrition" because pesticide, insecticide, toxins, plastic, and heavy metal contamination were not a part of our diet decades ago.

Here is another problem: even organic livestock still harbor dangerous toxins in their fat deposits.

Another issue is that livestock treated with antibiotics can damage our inner ecosystem, and this wreaks havoc including increased bad cholesterol as well as accumulation of excess body fat.

For these reasons, I recommend dishes containing high amounts of animal fat only until week 8 when we'll learn how to balance these tasty treats, but even then, you should eat them in moderation.

Which types of animal proteins are low in fats?

Poultry: Turkey without skin, chicken breast without skin.
Pork: pork chop.
Dairy products: cottage cheese, low-fat cheese, farmer's cheese (queso fresco) low-fat yogurt, low-fat kefir.
Cold cuts: Turkey ham, low-fat pork ham.
Fish and seafood: all types.
Beef: skirt steak, filet, veal.

Starting this week, you can choose any one of these low-fat proteins, but please do not eat beef daily. Remember to weight your 2 ounces of protein AFTER COOKING (except for cheese).

You should also moderate ingestion of large fish such as salmon and tuna and eat at most 12 ounces per week. This way you can reduce excess mercury load and toxic chlorine byproducts in your diet.

Animal protein should be cooked or grilled and prepared without butter or cream. Use cooking spray to avoid having your protein stick to the pan. Use cheeses with a low-fat content. There is a practical way of finding out how much fat is in a piece of cheese: If it does not melt when you heat it over a grill, it can be considered low in fat. But if it melts quickly, it may contain moderate to high amounts of animal fat.

Other types of animal protein will be used later in the program. And why will you be eating high amounts of animal fat if this might cause health problems in the long run? It would be naïve to believe that we will NEVER indulge in foods with large amounts of animal fat. A more sensible approach is to balance them to avoid body fat accumulation.

Perhaps a book recommending occasional use of bacon, goose, goat or lamb may be bland, but it's probably healthier. We naturally prefer foods with high-fat content, but in my day-to-day practice, I have confirmed that it is possible to develop and maintain permanent healthy eating habits so long as the total fat intake is lower than 35%.

Balanced Pack 4

For breakfast and dinner

2 slices of any bread (total 2 ounces – read below)

1 ounce of low-fat protein

1/3 of a medium-sized avocado, or 18 medium olives, any type

Lettuce, tomato, mushrooms, etc.

1 cup of cantaloupe, honeydew, papaya, watermelon, strawberries, or 4 ounces of any fruit juice

Calories	Carbohydrates	Total protein	Total Fat	Saturated Fat	Fiber
359	53%	17%	30%	8%	6 grams

This week, we'll have tons of fun with a meal that is very popular all over the world: the sandwich. You can eat it anytime, anywhere, and therefore I call it the "portable body shaping pack."

Use two slices of bread totaling two ounces. Which bread? It all depends on your preference, and lately, on the possibility of having gluten intolerance.

Gluten intolerance was uncommon years ago, but recently it has increased. It is hard to pinpoint where this problem is coming from, or what is causing it. But if gluten makes you bloat, you should REDUCE OR RESTRICT IT FROM YOUR DIET.

You find gluten in wheat and other grains, therefore a person with gluten intolerance should avoid wheat and wheat products in their diet.

By the way, up until this week, you have been on a low gluten diet! So be careful that you do not get bloated when adding wheat products.

If you suspect that you have a wheat intolerance, first use sourdough, which is made with wheat, but from the long-fermented dough.

Many people with wheat intolerance will tolerate sourdough. It is also absorbed very slowly, which helps people with diabetes obtain better control of their blood glucose.

If sourdough bloats you, try other types of bread that do not contain gluten, such as Ezekiel bread, and it should not cause problems. There are many gluten-free breads so do your homework when shopping.

Now, if you still get bloated after switching to gluten-free bread, go to your doctor; you might have gut flora imbalance, parasites, fungi, or protozoa. They all cause carbohydrate intolerance.

If you are one of the lucky ones that CAN eat wheat bread, then you have a lot of decisions to make.

The list of wheat bread to choose from is enormous: anadama, bagel, Bastone, beer bread, bhakri, bialy, bing, black bread, borodinski, rolls, ciabatta, Cuban bread, focaccia, matzo, multigrain, French roll, etc., etc., etc.

Just remember to eat only 2 ounces of bread.

Regarding your protein, it is a small portion. So, measure your ounces carefully. If you have cellulite, tuna packed in water is an excellent choice.

Use 1/3 of a medium avocado, which should weigh around 50 g. You can change the avocado for 18 medium olives.

Add tomatoes, onion, and peppers one day, mushrooms on another day, and even pickles on the third day. t will help you avoid getting bored with your sandwich. Change the type of bread you use.

Remember that you can use mustard, salt, pepper and hot sauce. To maintain dietary balance, avoid adding sour cream, butter, mayonnaise, etc.

The measuring cup of cantaloupe, honeydew, papaya, watermelon, and strawberries can be substituted with ½ a measuring cup of any other fruit (mango, apple, banana, etc.). You can also choose seasonal fruit– which is cheaper and tastier.

Instead of fresh fruit, you can have 4 ounces of fruit juice (freshly squeezed or bottled). Although freshly squeezed juice is preferable, if you don't make time to prepare it, buy bottled juice (apple, grapefruit, orange, grape, etc.) if there is no added sugar. Organic would be even better.

Now you have five different options for breakfast and dinner: Balanced Pack 1 (tostadas), Balanced Shakes 1 to 3, Balanced Pack 2 (oatmeal), Balanced Pack 3 (eggs) and Balanced Pack 4 (sandwiches).

Sandwiches are practical – they're fast to prepare, you don't need to heat them, and you can take them with you when you're on the go. You can even eat them while walking, or while you stand at the kitchen counter.

If you prepare your sandwich carefully, you'll obtain a satisfactory speed of fat loss. It's also very satisfying to know that you will lose excess fat even when you do decide to eat 4 in a day, although you will probably lose weight at a slower rate.

When you add new and more Balanced Packs, you increase the overall calorie count. But instead of obsessing over calories, focus on nourishing your body and enjoying your diet.

The advantage of all Balanced Packs is that if for whatever reason, you goofed and ate more than what you needed, you'll still lose weight and measurements. It might make you feel unpleasantly full, but this feeling will go away sooner or later.

If your imagination was larger than your needs and you ate too many Balanced Packs, you still have the unpleasant task of eating everything else indicated for the rest of the day, even when not hungry.

And if for whatever reason, you ate something outside of the plan (pastry, ice cream, cookies, etc.), you'll still have to eat the rest of prescribed meals in the program, exactly as they are laid out.

Balanced Shakes 1 to 3 are great go-to choices when you have gorged on something you shouldn't have and ended up stuffed. They make it easy for you to continue with prescribed meals.

WEEK 5

Basic Meal 5

Balanced Pack 5

Basic Meal 5

Early Morning: 2 ounces of 2% fat milk or plain low-fat yogurt
½ ounce or 4 saltine crackers (wheat or rice)
1 teaspoon of honey

Breakfast: Balanced Pack 1, 2, 3, 4, or 5

Mid-morning: 1 medium apple, banana, grapefruit, or orange
6 whole raw almonds or 3 whole raw walnuts
2 teaspoons of honey

Lunch: Fat-free vegetable soup
¼ cup of legumes: black, red, pinto, white, navy beans, lentils, or garbanzos (chickpeas)
2 ounces of low-fat protein
2 tsp. of olive oil, avocado oil, coconut oil,
or ½ medium avocado (80 grams of pulp)
1-½ cups of mixed greens salad
Water, tea, coffee (no sugar or milk), as needed

Mid-afternoon: **¼ cup of granola cereal**
2 teaspoons of honey
4 whole raw almonds or 2 whole raw walnuts

Dinner: Balanced Pack 1, 2, 3, 4, or 5

Late Evening: 2 ounces of 2% fat milk, or plain low-fat yogurt
4 crackers (wheat or rice)
1 teaspoon of honey

Calories	Carbohydrates	Total protein	Total Fat	Saturated Fat	Fiber
894	52%	17%	31%	6%	17g

Note: Foods in boldface increase total caloric intake from the prior week

Up till now, I have only recommended avocado and olives. Why? Because in my experience they promote greater fat loss than other oils but starting this week, you can also use olive oil or coconut oil for cooking.

You can divide fats into three groups: saturated, monounsaturated, and polyunsaturated. The body processes each of these fats differently.

The current recommendation is to reduce your intake of animal fats found in abundance among warm-blooded animals.

You find mono- and polyunsaturated fats in vegetables and cold-blooded animals. The current advice is that balanced diets contain around 20% of these fats.

Saturated and monounsaturated fats are very stable when they are submitted to heat, while polyunsaturated fats are usually not. High temperatures cause polyunsaturated fats to produce free radicals (molecules that severely damage the cells of the body, increasing the risk of arteriosclerosis, cancer, and premature aging).

Consequently, a healthy diet is supposed to have 10% or less of saturated fats, 10% or more of monounsaturated fat, and the other 10% of polyunsaturated fats, and even better yet raw vegetable fats (avocados, olives, almonds, walnuts and other nuts).

If your eyesight started to get blurry over what you just read, don't worry, the dietary guidelines mentioned above have been considered when preparing these programs.

In this new week, you will be able to cook your food with oil, but you must use one that is high in monounsaturated fat or saturated fat. These are extra light olive oil, avocado oil, or coconut oil.

Coconut oil is different from other saturated fats, and recent research has reported that it has some amazing health benefits.

First, it does not elevate the risk of having coronary disease or stroke. Second, it is minimally affected by heat, so it is an excellent choice for deep-frying (aka French fries and fried fish). Another benefit is that it is antimicrobial, antifungal and antiviral. The best one: not only does it promote weight loss; it also helps you to reduce abdominal fat preferentially! Oh, and I have also observed that it can contribute to cellulite reduction!

Do not switch out raw nuts that accompany fruits for olive oil, unless you are allergic to nuts. Why? Combining fruits with nuts may help you lose excess body fat faster. It could also protect you from developing diabetes.

Balanced Pack 5

For breakfast and dinner

2 slices of bread, one French roll, or 2 medium-sized corn tortillas (totaling 2 ounces), or 1/3 cup of steamed rice, or quinoa, or pasta

1 ounce of low-fat protein

½ of a medium-sized avocado, or 24 medium olives

¼ cup of beans, chickpeas, or lentils

Vegetables, as much as you like: red tomatoes, onion, lettuce, mushrooms, etc.

1 cup of cantaloupe, honeydew, papaya, watermelon, or strawberries, or 4 ounces of fruit juice: orange, grapefruit, apple, etc.

Calories	Carbohydrates	Total protein	Total Fat	Saturated Fat	Fiber
397	54%	16%	30%	5%	13 g.

This week, the servings method (see below) is used in Balanced Pack 5 to provide variety and flexibility.

2 ounces of bread (2 regular slices) have the same nutrients as 2 ounces of French roll or 2 ounces of corn tortillas.

Avocados, olives, and olive oil have similar nutrition content if you eat prescribed proportions.

Thanks to many similarities among different foods, they can be classified into different food groups. Let's look at these food groups:

Vegetables: chard, celery, watercress, red tomatoes, lettuce, radishes, etc.

Fruits: strawberries, mango, cantaloupe and honeydew, oranges, papaya, pineapple, banana, watermelon, etc.

Grains: rice, bread, pasta, corn tortillas, quinoa, etc.

Proteins: shellfish, beef, fish, chicken, duck, etc.

Fats: refined oil, olives, avocados, nuts, and seeds, etc.

Refined sugar: white sugar, sugar cubes, jellies, honey, etc.

Each food within the group is given a servings size so that their caloric value is similar.

This way of classifying foods into groups and giving them a serving value was proposed and accepted over 80 years ago. At first, dieticians used it to create diets for people with diabetes.

Nowadays, the food group system is used to create all types of diets for the healthy as well as the ill. It gives you the option of creating menus that are varied yet precise enough to generate excellent results.

It is relatively easy to calculate the approximate quantities of calories, carbohydrates, proteins, fats and fiber that we need for a nutritional system.

Although the method works, let's be clear that there are significant differences within each food group (and servings of foods within each group).

For example, corn tortillas have more calcium and fiber than bread. Moreover, even when pasta and sliced whole wheat bread are both made with wheat, pasta is absorbed much slower, which makes you feel full longer.

One tortilla is calorically like 2 cups of air popped popcorn, but popcorn fills us up more than corn tortillas: it is easier to eat six corn tortillas than 12 measuring cups of air popped popcorn, even when they both contain similar calories.

If we compare avocados, olives, and olive oil, we find that the first two also contain proteins and carbohydrates, while olive oil has no proteins or carbohydrates.

Legumes (black, red, white, navy, and pinto beans; lentils; and garbanzos) are considered proteins. However, their positive impact on excess body fat is so spectacular that if it were up to me, I'd give legumes their independent classification and serving sizes.

Balanced Packs 1 through 3 use specific nutrients to achieve a faster loss of weight and measurements. Balanced Pack 4 makes the program more practical, and Balanced Pack 5 uses serving size as a tool to enhance flexibility, even when weight loss may slow down.

Why add variety when there is a risk of creating a more gradual weight loss plan?

People have convinced themselves that it is all about gaining or losing weight and fat. They have forgotten that they used to eat whatever they wanted and still maintained a stable and healthy weight.

There is a huge obsession with slimming down, but the truth is that 90% of the time people are not following any weight reduction program because they are eating whatever they want. A telephone survey conducted in the United States demonstrated this.

In over 35 years of experience in treating excess body fat, I have realized one rule: when people force themselves to lose weight quickly, they get tired sooner or later, drop their plan, and return to destructive old eating habits only to regain whatever they lost, or gain even more.

In one survey, dieters ended up with 120% of their original weight after two years of dieting. Talk about extremely disappointing results regarding long-term weight loss outcome, right?

If you still want to lose weight quickly, even after knowing the disastrous long-term results and the importance of focusing more on habits than rapid weight loss, drop this book right now. Run to make an appointment with a psychologist or join a self-help group ASAP!

What combinations can you create with Balanced Pack 5? The sky is the limit!

Be creative, change ingredients, change spices and change your life!

Balanced Pack 5 can also be doubled, tripled, or quadrupled if you stick to parts.

During this week, you will use any of Balanced Packs 1 through 5. Remember that you can mix and match.

You can duplicate or triplicate these Packs at any moment of the day. You can double or triple them at breakfast and dinner, at mid-morning, at lunch, in your Mid-afternoon meal, or anytime you feel hungry.

Doubling dinner or breakfast is much more practical, but if you can set aside the time to eat a new Balanced Pack at any other moment of the day, you could achieve a faster loss of weight and inches. For instance, instead of eating six tostadas at breakfast at 8:00 a.m., you can eat two at 8, two at 10, and two more at 12 for better results.

If you're in a hurry to drop the pounds, or if you have issues with blood glucose, it is to your advantage to eat multiple small meals during the day.

Be very careful when doubling Balanced Packs, because you must still eat ALL foods from your Basic Meal. If you ate too much in the morning and you realized that, perhaps, EIGHT tostadas were a bit excessive, you will have to tough it out and eat everything else that is scheduled, even when not hungry!

Once you have mastered combining food groups into different dishes, you will have an incredibly powerful weapon that promotes the loss of fat around the belly button.

In the first four weeks, you learned how to reduce lower abdominal fat. This week, you will learn about three magical keys needed to eliminate fat loss around the middle part of your waist. Are you ready?

These are the three keys that open the door for a spectacular waistline:

1. A balanced diet.

2. Variety

3. Green-leafy vegetables in abundance.

Now let's review each one:

A balanced diet:

This is what you have been doing since Week 1. A balanced diet, as we stated earlier, has around 55% carbs, 15% protein, and 30% fats. These calories must be eaten in sufficient amounts to reverse and avoid Starvation Mode. If you are in Starvation Mode, it will be almost impossible for you to target specific areas of the body that you want to eliminate. If you have finally reversed Starvation Mode, you should start noticing how both belly button and lower abdominal fat begin to melt.

Variety

Our body needs all sorts of nutrients to work properly, and this includes carbs, protein, fiber and fats as well as vitamins, minerals, probiotics, and trace elements. Unfortunately, and in my experience, when you obtain vitamins and minerals through pills such as oral vitamins or supplements, you will not reduce waistline.

YOU MUST GET ALL YOUR NUTRIENTS THROUGH FOOD IF YOU WANT A SPECTACULAR WAISTLINE.

No single food will give you all the nutrients that you require. You need to eat a wide variety of foods to lose that unsightly tummy and turn it into a bikini-worthy waistline. This is what I want you to do during this week: eat a great variety of foods. You may very well be totally impressed by the results!

Green leafy vegetables

How this happens, I'm not sure, although I have a pretty good idea.

There is a form of fat mobilization that I have coined the FAT SURPLUS MODE, and it has nothing to do with fat loss obtained with traditional low-calorie diets.

It is my belief that when you have given your body exactly what it needs in sufficient quantities, it decides to eliminate fat because it is not required anymore. Our body is a very thrifty machine, and it will not maintain what it does not need. This holds true for enzymes, muscle, brain cells and even body fat.

This is the opposite of what happens with calorie-restricted diets since our body will use fat storages to survive. I call this fat mobilization the FAT DEFICIT MODE.

One of the fastest ways to generate "fat surplus mode" is to eat large quantities of green-leafy vegetables as well as all the other nutrients needed to obtain a balanced and sufficient meal.

It is very probable that signals sent through green-leafy vegetables instruct the body to utilize not only the fat within the cell but even the cell itself, i.e. WE START EATING OUR OWN FAT CELLS!

Amazing!

Some vegetable molecules even reduce blood flow to fat cells, which also causes the fat cell to be destroyed. This is another part of excess body fat research that is entirely outside of the scope of this book.

But don't worry about the research, because even if you do understand all the biochemistry involved, it will not work unless you EAT your veggies! Again, the solution is simple; eat large quantities of green-leafy vegetables!

I will tell you a beautiful (almost fairy-tale) story of one of the green-leafy diets which I developed: I created a balanced cold pressed vegetable juice diet with only 1,300 calories per day. And wow was I shocked with results!

First, if I want women to get firmer breasts, they need an entirely different approach (you will learn about it later) with at least 1,800 calories per day, and ideally more than 2,000 per day PLUS PASTRY.

I usually do not use diets with less than 1,200 calories, because they can cause loss of breast firmness and sometimes they can even sag terribly.

Well, it turns out that with this juicing diet that contained only 1,300 calories, my female clients not only lost waistline (that was the idea); they also reported firmer and even larger breasts!

This is exactly the OPPOSITE of what I see with my 1,300 calorie diets! Let me repeat it: I need to program at least 2,000 calories of a balanced diet per day to generate firmer breasts!

So where could they have possibly gotten those extra 700 calories of a spectacularly nutritious diet to create firmer breasts?

I believe that their bodies received signals from green vegetables to utilize fat cells and convert these cells into nutrients for a beautiful mammary gland.

Sounds impossible? Well, it sounds crazy to me too, but there is no other way that I can explain it.

Imagine, the body utilizing its own fat cells to rebuild other parts of itself. Will there ever be a special diet that specifically activates stem cells and lipid cells at the same time to work together and create new brain cells or new liver cells? It sounds wild, but only time will tell.

This information might blow the minds of not only the general population but also nutritionists, dietitians, doctors, and investigators.

And then again, if what you have just read doesn't make any sense, the solution is simple; if you do not understand what happens inside your body, it doesn't matter if you apply the rules.

You can use any green leafy vegetable, but try to include power greens. They are mustard greens, watercress, kale, turnip greens (leaves), collard greens, chard, spinach, and Brussel Sprouts. Just be careful to cook them so that it is easier for your body to digest. You can also juice them, and that makes it much easier for your body to absorb their nutrients.

Do not overeat kale, it can shut down your thyroid.

So, folks, happy hunting for that six pack or bikini waistline!

A word of caution: if you get lost when applying variety, go back to weeks one and two.

What can you do to avoid getting lost?

Plan what to eat for a whole week. Write everything down on a sheet of paper. Even if at some point, you decide to use something else (which you can and probably will), it doesn't matter because you have set in your mind an order. If you buy your supplies for the whole week, you will have even better chances of success.

It's like taking the training wheels off your bike and venturing without them.

Maybe you're even ready to take the bike on mountain trails!

Is it scary? Of course, it is.

Permanently losing weight and inches is not an easy task. I never said it was. I know very well through experience with my clients and myself that you might have to repeat the program two, three or four times before you obtain the "aha" moment.

And it is not that I want to scare you, just know that if you do get a little lost and maybe even feel panic, you are not alone in this journey.

Once I heard that action conquers fear. That has been my mantra for years, and that is what I want you to do. Get into action and keep on going even if you do have to return to weeks one and two.

WEEK 6

Basic Meal 6

Balanced Pack 6

Basic Meal 6

Early Morning: 2 ounces of 2% fat milk or plain low-fat yogurt
4 crackers (wheat or rice)
1 teaspoon of honey

Breakfast: Balanced Pack 1, 2, 3, 4, 5, or 6

Mid-morning: 1 medium apple, or banana, or grapefruit, or orange
8 whole raw almonds or 4 whole raw walnuts
3 teaspoons of honey

Lunch: Fat-free vegetable soup
½ cup of beans, or lentils, or garbanzos (chickpeas)
2 ounces of low-fat protein (explained in Week 4)
2 teaspoons of olive oil, or avocado oil, or coconut oil, or ½
medium avocado (80 grams of pulp)
1 ½ cups of mixed greens salad
Water, or tea, or coffee (no sugar), as needed

Mid-afternoon: **2 ounces of any type of pastry**

Dinner: Balanced Pack 1, 2, 3, 4, 5, or 6

Late Evening: 2 ounces of 2% fat milk, or plain low-fat yogurt
4 crackers (wheat or rice)
1 teaspoon of honey

Calories	Carbohydrates	Total protein	Total Fat	Saturated Fat	Fiber
894	52%	17%	31%	6%	17g

Note: Food in boldface is added in Basic Program 5 to increase total caloric intake

This week, we will add more almonds plus another serving of legumes (black, red, pinto, white, navy, or green beans, lentils, or garbanzos (chickpeas), and 2 ounces of pastry (yes!), representing an increase from 799 to 896 calories.

Congratulations! You've been on a unique nutritional program for a month and a half. Surely, you've already noted the following results:

- Less obsessing over food

- Elimination of the fear of eating

- Enhanced self-esteem

- Less insomnia and improved mental clarity

- Smoother skin and softer, shinier hair

- Less constipation, colitis, and gastritis

- Stronger nails

- Loss of excess fat

- Enhanced libido

You will have undergone some nonvisible changes as well: reduced "bad" cholesterol and triglycerides, uric acid and creatinine, as well as the better control of your blood pressure and blood glucose.

Eating in the manner set out in this book can seem impractical at first. If you work outside of your home (as most of us do), you must prepare your food at home before leaving and carry it wherever you go. However, you will find that it's more than worth it!

You may have had to limit your social life and traveling somewhat because it's not easy to get these foods away from home. But your desire to permanently lose excess weight will overcome any obstacle. If you've gone crazy in the past and engaged in severe restrictions (which goes against natural human nature), I'm sure this method will seem a lot more pleasant.

If this Basic Meal seems excessive, go back to one of the previous Basic Meals (1 through 5), which have fewer calories. You may feel more comfortable with Basic Meal 1 plus another of the Packs I've already presented. The most important thing is to feel satisfied, but not stuffed!

Balanced Pack 6 A

For breakfast or dinner

30 g (one serving) of processed cereal (110 to 140 calories)
8 ounces of 2% fat milk or coconut milk
4 raw almonds or 2 whole raw walnuts

Calories	Carbohydrates	Total protein	Total Fat	Saturated Fat	Fiber
270	55%	16%	29%	11%	3 grams

Meet a new Balanced Pack that's practical and tasty, although not the best nutritional choice. If you look at the fiber content, it is dismally low. And the table of Nutrition Facts is just ugh!

These processed cereals can be Cocoa Puffs, Captain Crunch, Cheerios, etc. The table of nutritional information will give you calories per serving which should be between 110 and 140 calories.

Which cereals are the healthiest? In all truth, that's oatmeal, but then again, processed cereals are way easier to prepare.

As a rule of thumb, check the Nutrition Facts and choose those cereals that have the LEAST extra ingredients such as artificial coloring, artificial flavors, etc.

Processed cereals with more calories (granola, Basic 4, etc.) or fewer (All-Bran, Fiber One, etc.) don't fit in this pack, not because they're unhealthy, but because they require different ingredients and quantities to be balanced.

Many people use fiber-rich cereals, and it is a good practice indeed. It encourages better digestion, can reduce cholesterol, may lower your risk of cancer, and last, but not least, it is pleasantly filling.

Here is a way to make your morning cereal a little healthier:

Balanced Pack 6 B

For breakfast or dinner

1/4 cup of fiber-rich cereal
30 g (one serving) of processed cereal (110 to 140 calories)
8 ounces of 2% fat milk or coconut milk
6 raw almonds or 3 whole raw walnuts

Calories	Carbohydrates	Total protein	Total Fat	Saturated Fat	Fiber
302	53%	17%	30%	10%	10 grams

High fiber cereals are original All Bran and Fiber One.

Many people are lactose intolerant (lactose is sugar found in milk and other dairy products). If this applies to you, or if you'd like some variety, you can switch out milk with low-fat kefir. If you still experience discomfort (gas, cramps, and even diarrhea), use coconut milk, almond milk, or rice milk. Nutrient content is indeed different, but when you add it to the rest of your diet, it is a good enough fit to encourage the loss of excess body fat.

Previous Balanced Packs have less than 5% saturated fat. They are aesthetically focused because, in addition to blasting body fat, they help reduce cellulite. Although cellulite isn't a disease, it does cause emotional distress. Patients notice that these packs reduce cellulite considerably.

This week you can enjoy a wide variety of options for breakfast and dinner: tostadas, eggs, sandwiches, and even cereals you used to enjoy as a kid.

Just remember that processed grains have a long list of extra ingredients that you do not want to add to your body daily. Use this Balanced Pack occasionally.

Remember that you can combine all Balanced Packs. If you're hungry, you can eat a sandwich PLUS a serving of "kiddie" cereal with low-fat milk and almonds. Just be careful with how your body reacts to the extra calories.

WEEK 7

Basic Meal 7

Balanced Pack 7

Basic Meal 7

Early Morning: 2 ounces of 2% fat milk or plain low-fat yogurt
4 crackers (wheat or rice)

Breakfast: Balance Pack 1, 2, 3, 4, 5, 6, or 7

Mid-morning: **2 slices of bread**
1 ounce of low-fat cheese
¼ medium avocado
4 ounces of fruit juice

Lunch: Fat-free vegetable soup
½ cup of beans, or lentils, or garbanzos (chickpeas)
3 ounces (90g) of low-fat protein (explained in the
previous chapter)
1 teaspoons of olive oil, or avocado oil, or coconut oil, or ¼
medium avocado (80 grams of pulp)
1-½ cups of mixed greens salad
Water, or tea, or coffee (no sugar), as needed

Mid-afternoon: 2 ounces of pastry

Dinner: Balance Pack 1, 2, 3, 4, 5, 6 or 7

Late Evening: 2 ounces of 2% fat milk, or plain low-fat yogurt
4 crackers (wheat or rice)

Calories	Carbohydrates	Total protein	Total Fat	Saturated Fat	Fiber
1053	54%	17%	29%	5%	18g

Note: Foods in boldface increase total caloric intake from previous Basic Meal.

I hope you enjoy the changes for this week.

The more foods you add, the higher the risk of regaining part of what you lost, and the reason for this is that you might still be in Starvation Mode.

Why would you still be in Starvation Mode?

Because you haven't done the program the way you should. As you will read below, making a perfect diet is QUITE DIFFICULT.

Dietary habits have lately received enormous attention.

For me, two studies are paramount for permanent fat loss, and you need to understand them well, and more importantly, accept them as part of your life.

These two studies apply to EVERYONE, including thin and overweight. There is no such thing as "I am different, this has nothing to do with me."

Once you understand and accept these studies, you will be on your way to recovery. If you don't, good luck trying to crawl out of a pit that is full of anguish, exasperation, disastrous diets, and more important, an unhealthy body.

The first phenomenon of altered eating habits is the following:

A group of people not on diet and a group who fasted for 24 hours were asked to taste six glasses of milk with varying fat content and were asked to choose which one was tastier. Both groups included thin and obese people.

Thin and obese people that were not fasting found milk with less fat tastier. The ones on a 24-hour fast preferred milk containing the highest amount of fat, and therefore calories.

Neither group knew the fat content of the milk they tasted.

Nutrient restriction, even if it is only for 24 hours, triggers an unconscious biological drive to eat products with a higher caloric content since high-calorie foods become far more appealing.

And if you did not register this information, the desire for high-calorie food holds true for BOTH THIN AND OBESE. All you must do is restrict calorie intake for 24 hours, and voila! High-calorie foods will become more enticing.

This drive to prefer a high-calorie food has nothing to do with all sorts of twisted explanations like lack of willpower, lack of self-esteem, an unconscious desire to be obese, self-defense mechanism, mother's fault for making you overeat, etc., etc., etc.

You can fill in the blanks with more biased explanations for overeating right here
_____ _____ _____.

I will repeat this again:

Restricting food intake will set ANYONE, thin AND obese, up for failure, because they will be spontaneously programmed to prefer high-calorie foods! It has NOTHING to do with thoughts and emotions.

This preference for high-calorie foods is one of many reasons why restricted diets will fail sooner or later.

Strict diets increase your probability to fail because they violate your natural drive to eat, and they unleash unconscious biological responses that push you to prefer high-calorie foods.

They also distort psychological and social patterns, but this complicated part of the equation is for another book.

And if this isn't enough, here is the other research that drives the last nail into the wooden coffin:

Thin and obese people were asked to carefully and obsessively write down what they ate during a whole month.

At the same time, they were injected with a radioactive substance to measure with meticulous precision how many calories they took during that month.

Results were surprising: thin people wrote down 20% fewer nutrients than what they ate. Obese under-reported by 40%.

It doesn't matter whether we are thin or obese.

Our conscious brain can only partly register what we eat throughout the day. The inability to consciously identify what we eat holds true even for those who carefully write down what they eat. If you have not been keeping a log, God only knows what went through your beautiful lips!

Limited awareness becomes even more so with excess body fat. Remember that obese were off by 40%.

We might believe that we are eating a 1,200-calories when in all truth, we are having over 2,000 calories per day!

Since we eat this extra food in total unconsciousness, it is impossible to know whether it is balanced or not.

And since we are restraining spontaneous food intake (that's what traditional weight loss diets are all about), these are most probably high-calorie high-fat foods. Do you remember the previous study?

I call this incapacity to recognize how much we eat the "PHANTOM ZONE."

We do not spontaneously register what we eat, but our metabolism certainly does! Even when we do not remember having eaten a slice or two or three of cake, our body still must digest it and decide whether to store it or burn it off.

You have eaten way more food than what you thought you did and are not even aware of doing it.

If what you ate in the "PHANTOM ZONE" was balanced, it helped you eliminate Starvation Mode. But it could have also happened that your unconscious eating, the "PHANTOM ZONE," reflected old, unstructured, chaotic eating patterns. If this was your case, it delayed the re-establishment of a healthy metabolism.

If you ate what you thought were enough Balanced Packs these weeks, you still took in 20% more of something else.

Fortunately, this is enough to reverse Starvation Mode, and you'll be able to continue with your weight loss while eating pastry and other delicious high-calorie plates.

But if you restricted your Balanced Packs because of fear of gaining weight, to lose weight faster, or perhaps because of stress, your "PHANTOM ZONE" most probably increased to 40% of a high-calorie unbalanced menu, and this might not have been enough to reverse Starvation Mode.

Have I confused you? If so, don't worry; accumulation of excess body fat is one of the most complex events of nature.

In a nutshell, if your weight and measurements go up in Week 7, it means you've only followed the program partially.

Eating extra food isn't as disastrous as it might sound, and you should not feel sad or guilty if you accept it and allow yourself to do the program better from here on out.

Toss your fear into the trash can and allow yourself to enjoy your food and eat as much as you want!

Balanced Pack 7

For breakfast or dinner

1 regular bagel of any type (around 105-gram weight)
1 ounce of regular organic non-diet cream cheese

Calories	Carbohydrates	Total protein	Total Fat	Saturated Fat	Fiber
369	58%	14%	28%	16%	2g

Who doesn't love a bagel with cream cheese?

Saturated fat content is high, and animal fat accumulates all types of toxins, so try using organic or grass fed cream cheese. Also, note how the fiber content is dismally low.

But then, naturally thin people can eat as many bagels as they want and remain thin, so if you've chipped away at Starvation Mode, you should be able to eat bagels one to three times per week and still lose weight and inches.

Milk has been getting an enormous amount of negative feedback lately, including the possibility of provoking cancer, increasing bone fractures, and increasing the risk of developing type 1 diabetes.

Perhaps these problems can be avoided by drinking organic or grass-fed milk. There is also another way of protecting your health: limit it to one glass per day.

Fortunately, cheese is not associated with these problems.

Aged cheeses can even reduce what is called "immune senescence" (immune deficiency caused by aging), and this, in turn, protects us from cancer cells.

So, cream cheese balanced with a bagel encourage a more active immune system, especially in the elderly!

What a fun way to better your health!

Just remember that you have at your disposal all the other balanced packs to work with, and that variety helps you reduce fat from waistline at a faster pace.

WEEK 8

The Plateau

Let's Have Fun!

Special Basic Meal

Early morning: 4 ounces of plain organic whole milk yogurt
2 teaspoons of honey

Breakfast: Balanced Pack 1, 2, 3, 4, 5, 6, or 7

Mid-morning: 1 medium apple, or banana, or grapefruit, or orange
6 whole raw almonds or 3 whole raw walnuts

Lunch: Special Balanced Packs (see below)

Mid-afternoon: 1 medium apple, or banana, or grapefruit, or orange
4 whole raw almonds or 2 whole raw walnuts
1 teaspoon of honey

Dinner: Balanced Pack 1, 2, 3, 4, 5, 6, or 7

Late evening: 4 ounces of plain whole milk yogurt
2 teaspoons of honey

AT LEAST 8 GLASSES OF WATER THROUGHOUT THE DAY

Calories	Carbohydrates	Total protein	Total Fat	Saturated Fat	Fiber
435	58%	12%	31%	11%	9g

4 ounces of plain organic whole milk yogurt with 2 teaspoons of honey are by themselves a Balanced Pack, which means that you can use this combination as many times as you want any time of the day! Just buy yogurt that has live active cultures. If you are intolerant to milk, try goat's milk yogurt.

Congratulations!

You've finished seven weeks of a tasty, balanced, and filling weight loss program.

You've already seen changes in your body, and your friends and family have congratulated you on your results.

Jokes and sarcastic remarks tossed around about your "crazy diet" have stopped, as well as any accusations that you are secretly taking weight loss pills. Some people even get accused of vomiting since they do not reduce their calorie intake. Talk about bias!

So, how much weight and volume will you have lost?

People experience a whole range of results, which depends on a series of factors:

If you started out the program with a bulging abdomen, i.e. with "metabolic lockdown," you probably noticed changes barely two or three weeks ago. Once the lower abdominal fat mobilizes, fat starts melting away in other parts of the body.

There are other possible scenarios:

You've used the program only for quick weight loss and have probably experienced ups and downs. Maybe a week ago you lost some, and then this week you gained some.

Maybe you changed from another diet after losing more than 20 pounds. You probably noticed minimal or no changes, and we will cover why and what to do in a moment.

If your previous diet caused severe malnutrition, you probably GAINED weight because of Starvation Mode and have just started to lose weight and inches one to two weeks ago.

Those with diabetes, high blood pressure, high cholesterol, triglycerides, major surgeries, and uric acid will lose weight and volume at a slower pace. Instead of getting a striking figure in a few weeks, the program generates a slow, safe, aesthetic reduction.

You could be one of those diet warriors who has been on strict diets, medications, supplements, and any possible treatment that you could lay your hands on. In this case, you must wait for your thrifty genes to shut down before your body starts changing.

Finally, you might believe that you have been eating an extraordinarily healthy diet because all your food is organic, you only eat vegetables, and you avoid all saturated fats and simple sugars.

That means absolutely nothing to your metabolism if your "healthy diet" was out of balance. Starvation Mode can be activated because you only ate vegetables and left out good quality protein and healthy fats and carbs.

With Starvation Mode comes an inability to lose excess fat, so you probably lost nothing at all or even gained some weight and inches during your first weeks of this free calorie program.

The average loss of volume is between three and five dress sizes in one to three months. Translated into body fat, you lose from 21 to 35 pounds of excess body fat, EVEN WHEN THE SCALE MIGHT SAY YOU HAVE LOST LESS WEIGHT. In this program, you reduce one dress size every time you eliminate around 7 pounds of excess body fat.

Those with more excess body fat will usually get more results.

Ups and downs are normal, and one week you might lose weight quickly, another week you might not lose anything or even gain a little.

Once you have lost 3 to 5 dress sizes or 21 to 35 pounds of body fat, you will almost always stop mobilizing fat, an event called the post-obese state. I prefer the other name which is PLATEAU, since many people are still obese after losing five dress sizes, and "post obese" seems a little off the mark to me. Here is another name if you want to research it on the Internet: diet resistant obesity.

Whatever you want to call it, the situation is the same: you stop losing weight and inches.

Even people with gastric bypass or gastric sleeve surgery hit plateaus, so guys; you are NOT going to dodge this bullet.

NOTE: Some fortunate people never hit a plateau and continue to lose excess body fat until they reach their ideal body weight and shape. I have seen this (which theoretically shouldn't happen) in less than 1% of my patients. It is so strange that I have sent all of them for a general checkup and thank God, all studies came back normal.

This event is so uncommon that if you are a dietician and have a client who never stops losing weight, please check with their doctor for diseases associated with weight loss.

So, what do you do when you hit a plateau?

You need to buy a beautiful, magical, mystical pill called PATIENCE.

Don't have any?

Well, you better get it any way you can.

Why?

Because if you try to force even more weight loss with severe dieting, supplements or medications, you will not lose any excess fat and might mess things up atrociously, generate Starvation Mode AGAIN, regain all the lost weight or even more, and go back to ground zero, or minus zero.

It makes no sense whatsoever, please, believe me, it doesn't.

And here is the good news:

After a period of "stagnation," which can last from 1 to 4 months, your body will start eliminating fat again.

How should the PLATEAU influence your behavior?

YOU MUST STOP TRYING TO LOSE WEIGHT AND INCHES.

The PLATEAU is a perfect time to forget your weight loss obsession because even if you make a deal with the devil, you will still not lose body fat for a while.

It is also the perfect time to add Special Balanced Packs, and I am confident that you will have tons of fun with them!

You should use Special Balanced Packs at most three to four times per week. I do not recommend them more often because saturated fat and heated oils are quite high.

In theory, this might cause damage in the long run.

Hopefully, your taste buds will have changed enough so that you notice how restaurant foods are not as tasty as home cooked food anymore.

Special Balanced Packs are the options to seek out in restaurants, or at homes of friends or family who are not following this plan.

Just like the regular Balanced Packs, Special Balanced Packs can be duplicated or triplicated. But be careful, because your body is not used to these foods anymore and they might cause abdominal symptoms. Healthy foods, if they are deep-fried, might also cause abdominal symptoms.

Life would be a little dry without all the yummy dishes such as pizza, hamburgers, French fries, chorizo, pork rinds, etc., right?

Can these foods be included in a balanced diet?

Of course, they can! Any food can be balanced.

Thin people do it every day: they eat these foods and stay lean. Some combinations are classic for thin people like pizza with a regular non-diet soft drink.

I call these Special Balanced Packs not because they are particularly good or special, but because you should use them on special occasions.

I want you to eat them at restaurants even when they are not the perfect place to recover from Starvation Mode. Why are they not the best place to revert Starvation Mode? Well, we do not know what oils they use, how long oils have been heated, and foods are usually not organic. They often use a lot of salts; some restaurants use MSG, we do not know how clean they are when preparing food, and they do not make food with the same love that you do.

Why would you want to add these Special Balanced Packs?

You need to know that you can eat these foods and stay thin.

Our body is a fabulous machine that was created to eat all sorts of foods, stay thin and survive. It is the ultimate survival machine.

If you eat at restaurants and maintain your weight and volume, you have recuperated the metabolism that you should have never lost, the one that keeps you lean if you avoid bad eating habits. You are now naturally skinny.

How should these combinations be used?

In my day-to-day practice, I recommend them under three circumstances:

First, as a self-test, so that you know just how your metabolism is working: I discharge my patients from the program when they can eat pizzas, burgers, etc. during a whole week and lose or maintain weight.

Second, to break up the routine a bit. Now and then, it's good to include foods that are supposedly fattening and see how excess body fat is still burned off.

Third, to mitigate emotional stress. You naturally crave high-fat foods when you're stressed out. That is why we call them comfort foods.

Instead of fighting this natural tendency, include them in such a way that they reduce Starvation Mode.

I have left out instructions as to how to prepare these Special Balanced Packs because you will be supposedly eating them at restaurants.

If you decide to make these dishes at home, you can "improve" them by using organic ingredients and coconut oil or extra light olive oil to cook them.

I have separated these packs into national cuisines. This should help you decide what plates to order depending on the restaurant.

So here are the Special Balanced Packs:

AMERICAN FOOD RESTAURANTS

Special Balance Pack 1

Small hamburger without cheese:

1 small plain hamburger without cheese

Calories 250

Talk about a defamed food that is balanced right off the bat! All you must do is eat it, and you can even add tons of ketchup and stay within the balanced range. Where do you buy this balanced meal? At McDonald's!

And since you can repeat any Balanced Pack, if one small plain hamburger is not enough, you just eat another one!

You cannot have French fries because they are not balanced. Well, you can, but you must accompany your French fries with other foods to maintain balance. Let's check this out:

Special Balanced Pack 2

French fries

One serving of French fries (74 grams)
8 fl. oz. of any soft drink
2 slices of nonfat American cheese

Calories 384

This Special Balanced Pack is a little tricky: first off, you only serve yourself 8 ounces of your favorite soft drink and second, you eat your two slices of nonfat American cheese when at home. Why at home? Because the cheese they add at the restaurant is not fat-free.

Can you do that?

Can you eat your Balanced Pack spread out over a 24-hour period? Yes, you can, and it works quite wonderfully!

It is not the most practical thing to do, and the greatest challenge is to remember to eat your two slices of cheese at home, but if you eat everything within a 24 or even 36-hour period, the body accepts this as part of a balanced meal!

It is what naturally thin people do, they balance what they eat today with what they eat 2 days from now, and do this in an entirely spontaneous way.

Talk about someone who is willing to forgive! It would be something like cheating on your spouse and getting the chance of making it right by not cheating within the next 36 hours!

Yeah, it's not going to happen, the concept of balance does not work on infidelity, ok?

And then there are other situations where balance does not apply: you are not only 0.1% pregnant. Either you are, or you are not!

So, going back to the hamburgers, soft drink, and French fries: you have combined two Special Balanced Packs and gotten away with murder (nutritionally speaking).

Is it healthy?

Wow, that is a tough question to answer.

If you take into consideration that these food combinations will promote the loss of abdominal fat (all balanced meals do), then it can be argued that it is a healthy choice since you are working to eliminate very dangerous body fat.

But if you consider ingredients, well, that's another story. I will make my bet that these combinations could harm your health in the long run.

You avoid these foods, not because they will make you fat since they won't, but because they are not your best choices.

Is there any way to make these combinations a little healthier?

Of course. At home, you use freshly squeezed fruit or fruit juice instead of soft drink, fry your French fries in coconut oil, use Himalaya salt instead of regular salt, use a sourdough bun and include grass-fed beef.

Is anyone getting a smile on his or her face?

I hope so. A delicious part of nutrition is how we relate to it, and I am not talking about calories. If thinking about food choices cherishes your soul, then my work has been worthwhile.

Special Balance Pack 3

McDonald's Quarter Pounder
Soft Drink or Fruit Juice

1-Quarter Pounder hamburger
14 ounces of regular non-diet soft drink or 12-ounces fruit juice

Calories 582

You are on the mark, since going to a restaurant to eat a plain hamburger is not that much fun. So, let's cheer things up a little bit with the way tastier Quarter Pounder that is not that close to a balanced meal, but you can solve by adding your regular non-diet soft drink.

Now, let's talk about soft drinks: It turns out that soft drinks made with high fructose corn syrup (HFCS) can indeed increase the risk of gaining excess fat. The risk of gaining fat with cane sugar is much lower. Bu then, where do you get these types of soft drinks in the USA? You don't unless you can buy bottled drinks made in Mexico. The European Union also sweetens their bottled drinks with sucrose. You lucky Europeans!

So, if you live in a country where soft drinks have HFCS, what do you do? Either you moderate, or an even better choice is to use fruit juice instead of soft drinks. The amount is a little less, 12 ounces.

And don't worry about the glycemic index (the speed at which the body absorbs sugar) since you are combining your fruit juice with protein and fats, and they put the brake on sugar absorption. So, fruit juices are an excellent choice when used at restaurants.

Which fruit juice is better? Research demonstrates how orange juice significantly reduces inflammation caused by restaurant food, so that would be your go-to choice.

If you decide to have fresh fruit instead of fruit juice, it's a lot! 12 fl. oz. of fruit juice is about to 2 small apples, or 2 pears, or 2 oranges. You may eat your other fruit at another time of day if it is too much for one sitting.

Special Balance Pack 4

Slice of Cheese Pizza, Thick Crust
Soft Drink or Fruit Juice

1 slice (about 3 ounces) of cheese pizza, thick crust
4 ounces of regular soft drink or 4 ounces of fruit juice

Calories 287

This is a very useful combination you can get nearly anywhere. However, before eating it for the first time, place a takeout order, bring it home, and weigh it out, so you'll have an idea of how much you're supposed to have.

You can eyeball the amount, and it is close enough for comfort. When you read the chapter on Weekend Extras, you will understand why you do not have to be obsessively perfect when measuring your Special Balanced Packs.

Special Balance Pack 5

Slice of Pepperoni Pizza, Regular Crust
Soft Drink or Fruit Juice

1 slice (about 3 ounces) of pepperoni pizza, regular crust
6 ounces of regular soft drink or 6 ounces of fruit juice

Calories 361

Not a bad combination. The caloric value does go up because you must add a little more soft-drink or fruit juice to balance the extra fat, but then you get to eat pepperoni on top of your pizza! And having a salad together with your pizza is also fabulous!

JAPANESE RESTAURANTS

Special Balance Pack 6

Salmon and Avocado Roll (sushi) with miso soup

1 Salmon and Avocado Roll
1 Cup of Miso Soup

Calories 382

It is another food combination that is balanced right off the bat!

It has all sorts of fat lowering ingredients: cold rice contains resistant starch, seaweed has tons of vitamins and healthy minerals (20 times more than the densest land plant), avocado consumption favors weight loss, and salmon has the omega 3 fats that are a rave nowadays!

And I cannot have enough praise for miso soup, which is one of the healthiest probiotic rich foods on the planet! The roll does not need miso soup to be balanced out, but calories do go down to 298.

Special Balance Pack 7

California Roll with miso soup

1 California Roll
1 Cup of Miso Soup

Calories 335

I added these rolls because they are very popular.

Fat and protein content is a little off. Therefore, we MUST add miso soup to make the combination work. You can find miso soup at any sushi restaurant.

Special Balance Pack 8

Caterpillar Roll with miso soup and almonds

1 Caterpillar Roll
1 cup Miso soup
12 whole raw almonds or 6 whole raw pecans

Do I seem biased by adding three sushi options? Not really, since the list is going to be long, but I'm happy to say that Japanese cuisine is a natural fit for any balanced diet.

You can add your nuts at any other moment of the day.

MEXICAN RESTAURANTS

Special Balance Pack 9

Beef, Cheese, Chicken or Pork Tamales with cooked beans

1 beef, cheese, chicken or pork tamale (total 110 g)
½ cup of cooked beans

Calories
326

This is a delicious and convenient pack that has helped a lot of people reduce their excess body fat.

I obtained the nutritional value from a Google search of different dietary data Web pages.

There is no need for a soft drink or fruit juice.

If you do decide to add a soft drink, you only need to drink 4 ounces plus 1 ounce of low-fat cheese (around 5 grams of fat per ounce of cheese). It increases the total value to 463 balanced calories.

Sometimes adding extras to your Special Balanced Packs can get a little tricky, but obviously, you can go for it.

Thin people do it naturally without having read this book, and you have all the hardware to do it also. We will be touching this fantastic news in the next chapter.

My advice, for now, is just to accompany your tamales with water until you become skilled at using these combinations.

Special Balance Pack 10

Sweet Tamales with milk, 1% fat

2 ounces of sweet tamale
1 cup of 1% fat milk

Calories
216

This is another delicious option; just keep the 1% fat milk handy when you get back home.

Special Balance Pack 11

Beef or Chicken Tostada
Soft drink

1 beef or chicken tostada
6 oz. of soft drink or fruit juice

Calories
221

Hmmm, the caloric value is quite manageable, so you just might decide to have ANOTHER tostada only to hit 442 calories, and you might still have space for a third one.

Ok, you just had your two tostadas: you did a lot of munching, and 12 ounces of soft drink or fruit juice is a nice amount. So just go slow with this one, and if you decide to triple it consider how full or hungry, you might be before your next snack.

12 ounces of soft drink or fruit juice have a lot of refined or simple sugars, but your body should metabolize them with ease. It is what we have been working for all this time. Just don't go crazy on your not so healthy drinks. Keep a calm head and maintain your Basic Meals and packages always at hand.

You should notice that soft drinks do not taste the same as before and that they tire you out quickly unless you are very, very thirsty. So, keep your thirst at bay with lots of plain water.

Since you have been eating a balanced diet, your soft drink craving should have dropped considerably. Why? Because you have been giving your body carbohydrates from all sorts of foods, so you don't need or crave pure sugar as much anymore.

Special Balance Pack 12

Beef, Chicken or Pork Pozole
Tostadas
Sour Cream
Soft drink

2 cups of beef, chicken or pork pozole
2 tostadas (fried in oil)
1 ounce of sour cream
10 oz. of soft drink or fruit juice

Calories
742

If you have never tried pozole, you are in for a treat!

Mexican pozole is a dish prepared with different spices, and it can be called Michoacán style, Jalisco style, or Guerrero style, but basic ingredients are the same for all of them.

You usually eat pozole with fried corn tortillas, and sour cream is added either to the pozole or on top of the fried corn tortilla. You MUST do that to balance out the pozole since its fat content is quite low. And since the carbohydrate content is also low, you must add either a soft drink or fruit juice to hit the sweet spot.

Consider the higher calorie count of this Special Balanced Pack. Your mind may not be conscious of what 742 calories mean, but your metabolism certainly is! Since you will be feeling full for some time, you can perhaps add a small fruit with nuts as your next snack.

Avoid adding "temptations" (extra food like pastry) to this pack, because it will likely turn off your appetite for 6 to 8 hours.

Special Balance Pack 13

Mole with Chicken and Rice
12 ounces of soft drink or 12 ounces of fruit juice

1 chicken thigh
½ cup of fried rice
1 cup of mole
2 medium-sized soft corn tortillas
12 ounces of soft drink or 12 ounces of fruit juice

Calories 764

Mole is a sauce that has been used in Traditional Mexican Cuisine for hundreds of years. It has all sorts of fat burning ingredients, and I would dare say it is the (better) American counterpart of Japanese sushi.

You might have to dig a little to find a Mexican restaurant that serves this sauce, but your search will be quite worthwhile.

Restaurants serve your mole with chicken, rice and corn tortillas; so, you don't have worry about bringing any of these ingredients from home! They're already there at the restaurant for your enjoyment!

DESSERTS

Special Balance Pack 14

Any Pastry
Low-fat milk
American Cheese (Nonfat)

A 2-ounce slice of any pastry
½ cup of 2% fat milk
1 slice of American cheese (nonfat)

Calories 278

I checked all sorts of pastry like chocolate cake, strudel, apple pie, pumpkin pie, cheesecake, pecan pie, donuts, as well all kinds of other goodies.

Pastries have a similar nutritional distribution, which makes balancing all of them feasible with the same foods, although I do accept that it is not a very practical option.

You do have to include that extra slice of American non-fat cheese, and your favorite restaurant will most probably not have it on their menu. So, you must add it at another time of day.

Not perfect, but we can have our cake and eat it too!

I understand that just 2 ounces are quite a small amount, but remember that you can duplicate or triplicate that slice of your favorite pastry if you accompany each slice with milk and cheese.

EVERYTHING ELSE

The list from the previous chapter is long, but in all truth, we are just scratching the surface of an enormous array of meals that we can add to our life.

I included the most popular dishes from Japanese, American, and Mexican restaurants, but each of these cuisines has a huge list of different plates that you can order. And guess what? I didn't even include them!

And we haven't even touched foods from China, India, Greece, Italy, France, Spain, Vietnam and so many other countries.

If you live in New York or Los Angeles, you probably think this is the most wonderful diet you have ever followed. It allows you to eat different foods available to you.

Ok, so let's set some things straight:

Although there is indeed a great variety of dishes that we CAN EAT, research suggests that we do not go past 20 different foods per month, and that is even a long stretch for many people. For example, most of us do not eat deer, bison, lizards, and insects.

So, immense variety is only an idea that does not reflect the way we eat.

We prefer what we ate since childhood: I seriously doubt that your mouth will water over guzzling down whale blubber and I don't think that an Inuit will kill for a papadzul (a traditional dish from Southeast Mexico).

Here is another thing: you can be incredibly creative and cook all sorts of dishes with the ingredients that you already have.

Even so, what do we do with such delicious but perhaps not so healthy dishes that have been left out? How do you solve this problem?

Should I create a list of combined foods so that you are always having a balanced meal? That would make for a huge book.

Perhaps I should create an APP where you can write in your grandmother's secret lasagna recipe, and it automatically programs the right foods that you need to add to turn that delicious lasagna into a balanced meal.

Or maybe I should create a HOTLINE where you can dial in, explain what you want to eat, and have the person on the other side help you choose what to add to make it a balanced meal.

That is what I did with a famous movie star, not because I had all the time in the world to do it, but because I wanted to know if it worked, AND IT DID!

She had just lost her husband, was going through a period of grief, and at the same time had to continue with a play that did not consider her husband's demise. She had stopped eating, and I knew that if this continued, we would lose all the work we had previously done together.

Since all she wanted was comfort food, I told her to call me and tell me what she was willing to eat. It was a happy ending for both of us! She ended up as beautiful as ever, and I got saved from being called a terrible nutritionist for leaving a major movie star either anorectic or obese!

Well, we do not have an APP or a HOTLINE at this moment, and fortunately, we don't have to! And here's why:

We can add disastrous dishes to our menu and stay slim!

Let me explain:

First, we must remember that our body is a fabulous survival machine and that it was programmed to identify nutrient distribution to decide whether to store or eliminate body fat.

We have already mentioned how thin people adjust their eating patterns in such a way that they consume varying amounts of food and generate balanced meals in a 36 to 48-hour periods.

Well, our body considers what we eat during ONE WHOLE WEEK, and if it is balanced, then it burns fat instead of storing it!

I see this in clinical practice, and it is what I use when people go on vacations since they eat whatever they want and still maintain weight and inches, or even lose some.

I used to send patients on vacations when on a 1,000-calorie diet, and they would gain huge amounts of weight and inches by the time they came back even when they tried to follow their strict diet.

Now I increase as many calories as I can, tell them to eat whatever they want every two to three hours, and they come back the same or even thinner.

You should be eating at least 1,350 calories daily before vacations, and the more, the merrier. It means that if you are on a 2,000-calorie balanced diet a week before holidays, it is almost impossible to gain excess body fat IF YOU EAT WHATEVER YOU WANT EVERY TWO TO THREE HOURS.

I call this the wave effect or wave phenomenon:

When a wave is coming into the beachfront and hits resistance, be it sand or rocks, it continues to advance because of all the energy it is carrying.

Something similar happens to people who go off my diets for a week and even for two or three weeks. They either maintain their body or even lose some fat despite eating whatever they want.

Isn't this fantastic?

You have been using a program that protects you from gaining excess fat EVEN WHEN YOU GO OFF IT FOR A SHORT PERIOD OF TIME.

I believe that our bodies even make decisions as to whether to accumulate fat or lose it depending on what has happened during the past month.

If for three weeks you have eaten in a balanced manner, and you have reduced Starvation Mode, then you can eat whatever you want for the fourth week without gaining any excess fat!

Obviously, there might be other reasons at play, and maybe one of them is that even though you are eating naturally, you are doing it as thin people do, i.e., you are spontaneously balancing all that you eat.

Whatever might be the cause, you still get a free pass!

This also happens if you add some disastrous dish at the end of only two weeks of a balanced diet.

So, if you are reading this and have already kept your diet for two whole weeks, you can add extra food in any one of two ways:

The first one is to eat whatever you want for a whole day, but you still must eat something every two to three hours.

Another option is to choose two meals to eat in a free manner during the weekend. It is the one most people want.

If you were disciplined with your meal plan during your previous weeks, you can eat whatever you desire on two occasions, be it breakfast, lunch or dinner, and continue to lose excess body fat.

You can go to a party, to a friend's house, or to a restaurant and eat whatever you fancy and still lose inches.

Isn't that just beautiful?

It takes care of hundreds and even thousands of meals. We do not have to balance all of them since they balance themselves out over time.

Well, that is not entirely accurate. Let me explain:

(A word of caution, you might get a little confused on the following explanation, but it is not necessary that you understand everything if you follow the rules).

Let's say that you are hitting 2,000 balanced calories during seven consecutive days. It means you eat a total of 14,000 balanced calories in a week.

So, you decide to add a disastrous plate, like eggs benedict, or eggs with hash browns, bacon, AND two buttermilk pancakes. Yum!

You have no idea how disastrously unbalanced these meals are, and I haven't even touched the percentage of saturated fats and total salt content. Believe me, it's bad.

When you add BOTH yummy breakfasts together and 24 ounces of orange juice to a nutrition software, it reports that on the AVERAGE you obtain 32% total fat, 8% saturated fat, 52% total carbs, and 16% total protein!!!!!!

It corresponds to a balanced diet and is, therefore, a fabulous result!

You can do it yourself if you do not believe me: download any nutrition software, add 14,000 calories of balanced meals and then add two disastrous meals plus 24 ounces of fruit juice (12 for each catastrophic plate). You will find out that these 16,000 or so calories are balanced.

And since these percentages fall within what the body considers a balanced diet, it will burn off any excess fat you ate plus whatever excess fat you have in your body.

There are some caveats to this situation, one of them that the higher your total caloric intake, the slower you burn fat, but you're still burning it.

There is another issue: if you can increase more than 1,000 extra unbalanced calories to your daily 2,000-calorie intake, you are messing things up quite badly. It is the perfect time to go back to the drawing board and check just what went on during your supposedly "healthy" week.

A person who is covering his daily needs in a balanced manner on a regular basis cannot possibly add 1,000 extra calories to his daily menu, he just can't.

It can only happen if he has been restricting his calorie intake for at least a week, or if he has not been balancing his diet.

Let's say you are eating 2,000 balanced calories per day, but your body needs 3,000: this means that you are on a 1,000-calorie deficit per day, and if this happens, you can easily add 2,000 extra calories on the weekend.

Ok, so you gorged on the weekend. What do you do? You INCREASE the number of Balanced Packs and a total number of calories during the next week since you have been eating less than what you need.

The extra meals that people add on the weekend are my way of knowing if I need to add more calories to their plan:
If they mention that they ate less of the usual amounts of their favorite cheat meal, then it means that I'm giving them what they need.

But if they tell me they ate disastrously and without restraint, then I must INCREASE calories to their menu. Since they are going to swear that they cannot possibly eat more, I add shakes.

The human mind is such a complex machine!

So, this is what you must do:

Consider that your two free weekend meals are a thermometer that will tell you how well you have covered your needs.

If you notice that hunger goes away even before you've finished your cheat meal, all is going well: what you are eating during the week is enough to cover your basic calories (yeah, that's what I call them, basic calories).

Just in case, don't force yourself to eat everything that is on the plate when you are not hungry anymore. Think about the following: you already paid for your plate. So, if you continue to eat beyond what satisfies your hunger, you paid to get fat! If you leave it on the plate, you paid to get thin.

The key is moderation: you are not adding a free meal to reward yourself for being such a good boy during the week. That is ridiculous!

You are adding unbalanced meals to learn to moderate them, and this is the key to permanent weight loss. This book takes care of balancing out your week. It is now your turn to eat unbalanced meals in such a way that they do not harm your body.

In all truth, you cannot honestly state emphatically that humanity "needs" chocolate cookies to survive. You really can't.

So, you should eat those foods that you do not need for survival in moderation. Do not eliminate them; they are not your enemy. Your enemy is overeating foods that you know are not necessary.

If you are ravenous when sitting at the table, and finish the plate while still wanting more, then hike up the overall calories of your weekly meal plan.

The freebie thermometer cannot be used to feel guilty about overeating. It is also ridiculous!

The freebie thermometer is just letting you know whether you ate less than what you needed during the previous weekend.

Why would this happen when you are trying to be a good boy or girl?

There are many reasons, and fear of food is only one of them. Perhaps all the fiber in your diet left you bloated, or maybe you have a gut bacteria imbalance that is inflaming your stomach or a stressful week that reduced your appetite, or you just could not eat because a family member ended up hospitalized, or you were sad because you got dumped.

Appetite reacts to so many external cues that it is incredible that more people do not have a weight problem!

So, don't beat yourself up for gorging on something on your freebie, since you have a whole new week to make things right. Our body is very forgiving, and there is nothing you can do with food to damage yourself in such a way that you cannot reverse it with a balanced diet.

Here is a very simple way to increase your caloric intake:

Remember the smoothies from Week 1, i.e. Balanced Smoothies 1 to 3 on pages 53 and 44?

Add at least one per day, and if necessary, as many as needed so that you get to your next weekend full and eat "freebies" without going crazy.

And now, ….

You are going to read my favorite chapter of this book, and it is the chapter about cravings!

CRAVINGS

This book would be incomplete without a section about cravings.

This chapter might generate confusion to some people, but remember that if you do not understand all the information, the solution is simple, just follow the instructions. Ok?

Recognizing and honoring your cravings is the ONLY way that you can forever get out of your diet prison. If you don't lose weight eating whatever you crave, you are doing something wrong, because when you are honoring your cravings, you WILL lose weight.

Let me explain:

First, cravings are crucial biological events.

Even when the mind and emotional and mental cues influences cravings, you must never discount them as merely secondary to an emotional response. If you make this huge mistake, you are putting yourself back into prison and losing the keys to the lock!

Cravings have huge biological foundations:

Our body needs different types of nutrients, and that is the fundamental reason we identify the desire to eat them. Think about it; we do not feel the desire to eat a cotton shirt, no matter how hungry we are.

The body translates a biological need for a nutrient into desire, and when we identify this urge (craving) with precision, we provide our body exactly with the nutrient it needs in the exact amount needed.

When our body runs low on sugar, we perceive a desire to eat something sweet.

When our body needs fats, we will crave something deliciously full of fat.

When our body runs low on protein, it asks for protein and not for sugar or sweets!

When we identify and fulfill these biological needs, our body rewards us by releasing endorphins and this, in turn, fills us with pleasure.

I call this an act of love: when we pay attention to our body and give it what it needs, we obtain an intense sensation of well-being.

But if we give our body something it does not need – or on the contrary, withhold what it needs – it is impossible to obtain this sensation of gratification or pleasure.

If our body requires sugars and fats, and we give it a piece of pastry, we find great pleasure from eating it.

But if on the contrary, we are extremely thirsty, and we eat a piece of cake, we're not gratified until we give our body the water it needs. We might even get angry for not receiving water!

A slice of pastry eaten at the wrong moment can generate a very unpleasant sensation. If you don't remember what it feels like to eat something that your body doesn't need, it's because you have been starving it for too long. Once you have deactivated Starvation Mode, you will often be telling yourself "oops, I didn't want that."

The number of calories we eat, as well as the type of calories we eat, are regulated with such spectacular precision, that it is ALMOST impossible to gain weight if we do not go into Starvation Mode.

How good are we at giving our body what it wants? We are incredibly accomplished, but only before the age of 6. Children who are less than six years old eat perfectly balanced meals. They have no prior knowledge of what a balanced diet is or is supposed to look like.

Now, the story changes after six years, because we start eating what we are EXPECTED to eat, and not so much what we WANT and NEED to eat.

Most children over six years of age will lose their spontaneous ability to balance a diet. And this lost ability will continue into adulthood.

You need to revive your childhood ability to identify cravings with precision, so that the next time you decide to put something extra in your mouth, it will generate a balanced diet!

How difficult is it to restore that ability? It should not be that hard, but you do have to throw all your previous ideas about what a "healthy" balanced diet consists of into the trash can.

They also call it "mindful eating," and it works quite well. You can look it up on the Internet, just don't get carried away buying tapes, DVD's, having hypnosis therapies, etc.

All you need is to restore something that is already yours, but you are so scared of your body, that you ignore it.

Isn't that ridiculous, to be afraid of your own body?

And the sad truth is that this fear is based on the fragmented and fallacious information.

Focusing only on weight is wrong, changing your food choices depending on what happens to your weight is wrong, severe dieting is wrong, fear of food is wrong, feeling guilty when you eat is wrong, Ugh!

And my question is not WHY all this happens; it is WHERE are you guys are going to draw the line?

To help people identify cravings more precisely, I have divided cravings into three different types. Each one has a function.

They are the following:

Mental cravings:

Mental cravings relate to our current lifestyle as well as our upbringing. Social norms shape it on top of biological needs. For example, it would be hard for an American child to crave yak milk, but children from the Himalayas who grow up on it will certainly find it entirely appetizing.

Mental cravings are not actual biological needs, although they can be.

Let's say that you are watching the Super Bowl, and a commercial about burgers comes on. You were not wanting or needing a burger, and you don't have one in front of you, but when the ad comes on, it suddenly entices you so much that your mouth even starts to water!

It is so common that we even joke about it: about how we are getting ready to eat cake at the birthday party, to enjoy pancakes at your favorite pancake restaurant, to eat some guacamole watching the Super Bowl, etc.

It happened to me when writing this book: while trying to figure out how to write this chapter, I woke up craving eggs benedict!

I was a victim of my mind! And what do you think I did that morning? Did I eat them, or did I avoid them? You will find out in a minute.

I will dare say that 100% of people on traditional restrictive diets will fall prey to mental cravings. Mental cravings can destroy even the best-planned weight loss program.

So, what do we do with mental cravings? Do we ignore them? Do we give in to them?

Here's the problem: a mental craving MIGHT be the reflection of a biological need.

And if it is truly a reflection of a natural need, you will generate fat loss when you eat it. Why? Because you will be covering a need as well as balancing your diet, and this shuts down Starvation Mode.

If you DON'T EAT IT, this could lead to an unbalanced diet, Starvation Mode, and accumulation of excess body fat.

Now, if you give in to your mental craving and eat something that your body didn't need, you are generating an unbalanced diet, and this will increase fat accumulation.

What a mess!

We cannot ignore it, and we cannot indulge in it.

What do we do?

We call in the cavalry!

When a mental craving appears, our next step is to ask another two regions of our body whether this desire is due to a basic need or not. These areas are lips and upper abdomen.

I have separated cravings into two categories: the first is water and sugar and the second one is protein and/or fat.

Water and sugar will be determined by what your lips communicate to you.

Protein and fat will be determined by what your upper abdomen tells you.

If either your lips or your upper abdomen confirms that your body needs a mental craving, then have it!

Going back to my eggs benedict craving, I first asked my upper abdomen if it wanted those eggs. Since my body said YES to the Benedict, I ate what my mind initially desired!

Let's see how this works:

Lips cravings:

Touch your lips with the tip of your fingers, and ask them if they want water or not. If you have a need for water, your lips will send the signal of thirst. They will immediately tell you that you need to go for some.

Are you feeling thirsty, now that you've touched your lips? Well stop reading the book and drink a glass of water!

Why are over 80% of adults chronically dehydrated? It is because they stopped listening to their biological signals.

Your lips also tell you how much water you need to drink: when you are re-hydrated, the sensation of thirst in the lips will disappear.

Your lips crave water because the body requires it, and you can identify a desire for plain water, fresh fruit, a soft drink, shaved ice, or coffee with or without sugar.

It means that your lips can ALSO identify your needs for carbs and even what kind of carbs your body needs.

There are all sorts of carbs in nature. We might not consciously know the difference between these different carbs, but our body certainly does.

When our body craves the carbs contained in a banana, it will crave just that.

Try it out. Ask your lips if they crave sugar and if your lips say YES, ask them what kind of fruit they want. The response is excellent! Sometimes they may even say: "No I do not want any fruit, I want honey!"

Hmmm, my lips just told me that they want a tangerine! And OF COURSE, I just ate one!

Don't ask your lips to identify the need for protein and fat.

If you want to know whether your body needs a piece of chocolate cake, or a piece of chicken, or an apple pie, ask your upper abdomen.

Upper abdomen cravings:

To identify your stomach cravings with precision, you must follow six rules:

One: Say hi!

Bring your left hand to the region that lies just below your sternum and say "Hi!"

Two: Use sweet sounding words.

Talk to your stomach with tenderness and love, as if you were talking to a small, wonderful child. Use affectionate words, and you'll sense its answer. You might even notice how you find a smile on your face! Just be careful to avoid harsh or insulting words, since you are in fact, talking to a beautiful part of yourself.

Three: Be patient.

If you receive an immediate response, it's your mind talking to you, and you should ignore it. You need to give your stomach at least a minute to make a choice, so wait patiently and quietly, and if your body does need something, it will surely let you know by way of a craving.

Four: Cravings have a first and last name.

Nobody craves a "carbohydrate" or a "protein." You want specific food with high precision. Cravings have a first and last name.

For example, fried chicken, blackened salmon, chocolate cake, Oreo cookies, etc.

Once your stomach identifies a desire, ask it to give that craving a first and last name: wanting any cookie is not a craving, but chocolate cookies are. So are oatmeal cookies, Oreo cookies, etc.

If you "crave" any cookie, it is not a craving; it is hunger. Non-specific needs appear when you are hungry. Hunger and cravings are two entirely different animals. Hunger is non-specific; it causes pain or discomfort and is accompanied by irritation and even with anger.

Cravings are accurate, the expectation of eating them brings pleasure instead of pain, and these needs come with a sense of excitement instead of irritation and anger.

If it has a first and last name, it's a craving. If it doesn't have a first and last name, it's hunger.

Five: You cannot bribe cravings.

Once you've identified your need and know its first and last name (for example, rocky road ice cream), try bribing your body with alternatives that are like what you want.

For example, if your body said rocky road ice cream, try to tempt it with strawberry sorbet, or with a vanilla ice-cream sandwich to truly identify the craving.

If you've identified your craving, your stomach will insist on exactly what it wants to eat. If you haven't yet determined what you want with accuracy, you should start the process over to define what your body is asking for.

Ok, your body tells you that it could enjoy lemon sorbet or rocky road ice cream. Your next step is to ask it to decide which one it wants the MOST. Once your body decides, you will notice that you cannot change it, no matter what other tasty dishes you offer, and no matter how much you insist.

This ability to define your cravings is so impressive that your body even tells you exactly how much it wants of that craving.

Depending on how your internal dialogue works, you might "see" the exact amount on your plate, while others might "hear" what portion they need and others will "feel" how much they should eat.

Six: Test it!

You obtain final proof when you take that food into your mouth. If you have a defined sensation of intense pleasure, you listened carefully to your body and gave it exactly what it needed to work optimally.

But if you do not enjoy that food, do not continue eating it, even if you already paid for it. Consider that you are paying to slim down.

When a dish not included in this book comes knocking at your door, first confirm that it is lips or stomach craving and not a mental desire.

Once you've learned to identify your desires with precision, you've won half the battle.

A word of caution: many things can hamper your ability to identify cravings.

The greatest one is malnutrition/under-nutrition. So, before going off to determine and fulfill carvings, please use at least two weeks of balanced meals first.

Cravings can also be muddled by physical and mental fatigue, lack of sleep, dehydration, acute and chronic stress, as well as intense emotions such as fear, anger, jealousy, contempt, exasperation, and many, many other emotions. Even love and lust go on to this list.

So, if you are going through an intense moment in life, ignore your cravings and make certain that you eat enough balanced meals to avoid Starvation Mode.

But the most common reason you cannot identify your cravings with clarity is that you have forgotten the ability. If there is one thing that traditional diets do, it is to forbid cravings.

So, in your attempt to get out of a deep hole, you have dug yourself in deeper. Recuperating that ability will take time, maybe even months, but if you work hard at it, you will recover this innate ability sooner or later.

The second most common reason to not identify your cravings is dehydration. Towards the end of a meal, you will sometimes feel that you are full in the stomach, but not on your lips. If this happens, take a tall glass of water and wait. It will solve the problem, and you will identify what it is that you need to eat more of, or your lips craving will go away.

Sometimes you know that you are craving something, but it is hard for you to identify it. Drink a tall glass of water even if you do not feel thirsty and this will help you identify your craving.

If water does not help you, ask your stomach whether it wants something salty or sweet. Just remember: you identify sweets without protein and fat with your lips.

If your stomach says it wants something sweet, offer your belly something that has sugar plus protein and fat such as a cake or a cookie. The same goes for something salty: offer your body a burger, a pizza, some chicken or shellfish, etc.

The further away you are from Starvation Mode and fear of food, the easier it will be for you to identify your cravings. But you do have to practice, and practice and practice.

NAVIGATING ROUGH WATERS

Excess body fat is one of the most complex phenomena in nature. It is no wonder that many people feel as if they were navigating turbulent waters in a rudderless boat at the mercy of wind and waves.

As if the complexity of this event wasn't enough, there are thousands of pages of contradictory and confusing information out there.

Should I cut down on my sugars, restrict my fat intake, or both? Should I eat only fruit in the morning? Can I eat refined sugars? What food combinations are the best, the ones recommended by Dr. Sears, or by the AHA, or the Asian diet, or the Mediterranean Diet?

This messy subject should be quite easy to solve: if some book recommends you eat less, you're doomed to fail.

Then there's part two of the puzzle: you read a weight loss book that says that eating less will not solve the problem, that you need to eat more to lose weight, but then it goes on to give a diet that is restricted.

This one is a little trickier since you get drawn in by theory, but in the end, the advice still boils down to food restriction.

I even got pulled into this trick by an internationally known diet book, but when I checked the diet program with a nutrition software, it turned out to be yet another calorie-restricted diet.

You don't have to buy a nutrition software to analyze all the diets that you read about (although you can). Just check to see if there is a chapter on cravings. If there isn't, they have just not gone far enough in their search for a permanent weight loss solution.

And do not even consider the idea that just by reading this book you`re out of the woods because you're not.

You will still be facing many challenges; your first one will be to wrestle with your internal dialogue.

About this, I'd like to point out something I find quite interesting. First, almost everyone bitterly complains about how slow my weight loss program is. However, when I ask them to compare it to other programs, they recognize that it's the most logical and fantastic one they've tried in their lives.

How can something be fabulous and frustrating at the same time?

I believe that this is because we use different criteria for measuring the events that affect our lives.

One is logical; the other (which usually rules) is emotional.

From a logical standpoint, we can understand that this method is a rational approach, and perhaps the only one worth choosing. From a psychological perspective, we find it sad (or frustrating, or exasperating, or whatever) to lose weight so slowly.

What do I do when strong wind and waves affect my journey?

To help you stay on course and make your voyage easier, I'll show you a routine that can keep you on track.

The mirror

You will need a naked body (your own!), a full-length mirror and 3 minutes of your morning. Once you have all three, you need to make a detailed inventory of your body:

Hair: Make certain that your hair keeps, or recovers, natural shine, a silky texture and good volume.

Facial wrinkles: Is your face starting to look like it's soon going to need Botox? Pay close attention to wrinkles around your eyes and your lips. Here's the good news: the program in this book usually make you look at least ten years younger! i.e. it reduces wrinkles!

Cheeks and lower jaw: If you have puffy cheeks and a "double chin," you should notice that they both disappear without leaving any sagging skin behind.

Neck: Make sure that the skin of your neck does not start to wrinkle or sag.

Arms: Hold them out to your sides, and check whether skin under the arms starts to fall or not. Some people even call this sagging skin "bat wings."

Chest: this is for women; stand in front of the mirror with your shoulder blades pulled back. Now identify where your nipples are pointing. They should be symmetrical, and both are facing forward. If they are not symmetrical, check daily to make certain that they do not get any droopier. You should also touch your breasts and confirm that they are not losing firmness. If they are sagging from the start, the program should help you obtain firm, youthful looking breasts.

Abdomen: make sure your stomach does not begin to droop, or if it is already sagging, that it doesn't do it even more. If you turn sideways, you will find it easier to identify what is happening with the lower part of your abdomen.

Glutes: Do you have a firm, toned, beautiful butt? If not, it's because of severe dieting, and not because of bad genes or age. You should not lose firmness, and if it is sagging, it should become firm and toned.

Thighs: do you have slim legs, or do they have excess fat? If they do, this must disappear leaving very sexy legs behind.

Calves: this should be the last part of your body to go down. Even though you might hate your thick calves right now, you do not want them skinnier, since this means that you are losing muscle, and setting yourself up to recover lost fat.

Skin: It should remain smooth and glowing.

I hope this routine mitigates negative emotions about slow weight loss. Hopefully gaining a more beautiful body will bring you more pleasure than a quick weight loss diet. Now, if your body is looking better and you are still unhappy and impatient with it, maybe it's time to seek emotional help.

In all truth, you seldom need fast weight loss, unless you have severe physical impediment caused by excess weight. Need for rapid weight loss is more related to poor self-esteem, and a beautiful body is seldom enough to increase self-esteem. Don't waste your energy and time that way. Look for other ways to increase your self-worth that do work.

Now, it is entirely possible that the first couple of times you may be shocked by what you see in the mirror. Some people even break up in tears.

But think about it, if you are surprised by what you see in the mirror, your body was that way yesterday and the day before.

Even if you find your body unappealing, carefully check those parts you DO NOT WANT TO LOSE or perhaps even want to increase to look better. Loss of excess body fat cannot be only about losing something; you must become ambitious and strive to GAIN something, i.e. a beautiful body.

I always tell my clients on their first visit that we will be shaping their body, and they give me a blank stare. After a couple of weeks, when they start noticing curves and tone, they finally grasp the benefit of losing excess body fat by eating more.

Our goal is to reverse Starvation Mode and recover or obtain the beautiful body that God gave us. It is not to lose weight as quickly as possible.

This program – or any other program, for that matter – is useless if instead or reversing Starvation Mode, you worsen it.

And no matter what program you use, you are always at risk of eating less than what your body needs.

Let your figure guide you in the best direction possible. If you use the routine I have described, you'll obtain these benefits:

First, it will help you stay focused on your plan all day long, giving you greater discipline and faster results.

Second, it will help you accept your body. Although it seems incredible, most people are ignorant of their bodies, and the mirror helps them recognize who they are and what to solve.

Third, it will let you know when you are eating too little. If you identify negative changes, such as a sagging breast, you know for certain that it is time to add more Balanced Packs.

Lastly, toward the end of the program, when you have obtained a new, more youthful and aesthetically pleasing body, you will have a powerful reason to continue.

When you finally look how you want, motivation to stay on track will diminish. From this point on, your goal should now be to maintain a young, firm, attractive, and healthy body.

Can the routine increase your vanity? I hope so. If vanity fuels your motivation, you will have still achieved benefits for body, mind, and soul by reversing a terrible problem.

Recommend this routine to friends or family members. You will be giving them a powerful tool that will them obtain better health. It will also assist them to steer clear of diets that do more harm than good. It is hard to find a program that makes you look better naked than with clothes on!

Expect your judgment to be entirely arbitrary the first couple of times that you check your body. It is normal: one day you might think you're looking awesome and the next an absolute mess.

All this will depend on the mood you're in when you wake up. Therefore, you should do it daily, for repetition lessens passion and heightens objectivity. After the first week, you can do it once a week.

You can use the chart that you will find on the next page to keep track of what you see in the mirror. Please make copies of these charts to keep a log of what is happening to your body.

WEEK ONE

	Sunday	Monday	Tuesday	Wednesday	Thursday	Friday	Saturday
Hair							
Face							
Cheeks							
Neck							
Arms							
Chest							
Abdomen							
Hips							
Thighs							
Calves							
Skin							

WEEKS 2 TO 8

	Week 2	Week 3	Week 4	Week 5	Week 6	Week 7	Week 8
Hair							
Face							
Cheeks							
Neck							
Arms							
Chest							
Abdomen							
Hips							
Thighs							
Calves							
Skin							

You can use the following symbols:

Looks good:	+
Better than before:	√
Worse than before:	---

Taking Measurements

A more scientific yet complicated routine is anthropometry, which involves taking measurements of your body. For this method, you need a measuring tape, your naked body, and lots and lots of practice.

The program outlined in this book causes a gradual loss of volume that is almost impossible to identify. In fact, over 90% of my patients come in complaining about how their bodies are not responding when in fact they have lost excess fat.

I've known very few people who can identify what, where and how much they have lost without taking measurements and without having to check the mirror. They are almost always high-performance athletes.

The rest of us mortals –myself included – require tools: a mirror, a measuring tape, some photograph or clothes that didn't fit anymore, to be able to identify changes in our body.

Therefore, it is essential that you use objective evidence. It includes, but is not only limited to what you see in the mirror.

Weigh yourself, measure your circumferences, take pictures, observe your body in the mirror, try on clothes that didn't fit before and keep a log of all these changes.

The exact area measured is not as important as measuring in the same place every time you do it.

These are the circumferences I take, being careful to have the measuring tape parallel to the floor (a mirror will help):

Arm: half way between the elbow and shoulder, with the arm extended to the side.

Breast: the measuring tape goes over both nipples. Women should ideally measure their breasts without a bra.

Chest: under the breast at the bottom part of the sternum.

Waist: the narrowest part of the waist, which is usually halfway between the bottom of the sternum and the belly button, right under the lowest part of the rib cage.

Umbilicus: over belly button

Lower abdomen: halfway between the umbilicus and pubic bone.

Hips: the measuring tape goes over the largest part of both glutes and in the front, over the pubic bone, unless the lower abdomen is hanging over the pubis. In this case, I am careful that the measuring tape is parallel to the floor.

Thigh: measuring rape goes right under the groin and over any bulges that might appear on the outer part of the leg. This measurement is seldom parallel to the floor.

Calf: I take multiple measurements until I find the largest circumference possible.

The very first time you do it, take THREE MEASUREMENTS AND take the average of all three. With practice, you will be able to be precise with circumferences.

A word of caution: it must be done by the same person because everyone measures differently.

This task must be carried out daily for at least two consecutive weeks. After that, you can do it once a week.

You can write down your results in the following table (in cm although you can use inches):

Day	Arm	Bust	Chest	Waist	Abdomen	Hips	Thigh	Calf
1								
2								
3								
4								
5								
6								
7								
8								
9								
10								
11								
12								
13								
14								

Week	Arm	Bust	Chest	Waist	Abdomen	Hips	Thigh	Calf
3								
4								
5								
6								
7								
8								
9								
10								
11								
12								

Below is a picture of the sites where I take measurements from my patients:

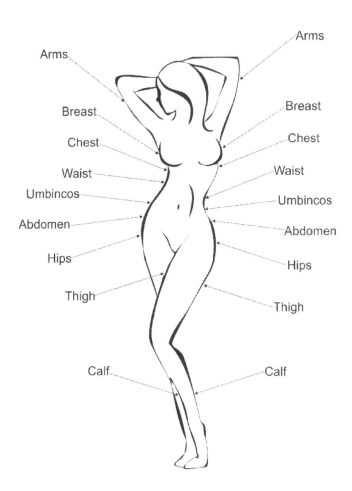

How to interpret changes:

Breast: When this circumference goes down, you are losing fat from the chest and breasts. If you are a woman, make certain you are not losing breasts. A loss of fat from breast leads to "rebound effect," which means you will gain back what you lost or even more.

Confirm that your nipples stay exactly where they started in the first place. Nipples that begin to sag are indicating that you are losing structural fat, which you shouldn't. If you are losing breasts, it is critical that you increase the number of Balanced Packs, EVEN WHEN YOU HAVE BIG BREASTS to avoid sagging. Here is some fantastic news: nipples that are already sagging will almost always go back to their original place with this program!

Chest: This circumference goes down when you eat something every 2 to 3 hours. If your chest stays the same, it means you are not eating as often as you should. Be obsessive about eating on time, and use your cell phone alarm to remind you to stop whatever you're doing to eat.

Waist: Fat around your waist is tightly tied to a variety of deficiencies, usually fruits, vegetables, and legumes, although insufficient fats and proteins also influence it. If your waist stays the same, you are consciously or inadvertently eliminating some element of the program.

Measure out food portions correctly, and if you are ever in doubt, add a little bit more. If you have a 25-g slice of cheese and a 35 g of cheese, choose the second one. Do you consider that you measure portions to perfection? Then add as many green leafy vegetables as you can.

Lower Abdomen: If you are not losing in this area, it can be one of three things: an unbalanced diet, a lack of soluble fiber, and/or intense and chronic persistent stress.

Weeks 1 and 2 were designed to take care of this region. If needed, repeat them again and again until you see changes. Remember that the rest of the body will go down very slowly if you have excess lower abdominal fat.

Increased amounts of fiber, irritable bowel, and/or parasites can cause abdominal bloating. This makes it difficult to know whether you are losing lower belly fat or not. If you have, or suspect that you have irritable bowel or parasites, talk to your doctor so that he or she can give appropriate treatment. It also helps to measure this body part early morning when bloating is usually at its lowest.

If after doing all this you still don't see the lower abdomen go down, seriously consider seeking help to lessen stress on your life. Perhaps you need to add to your diet psychological counseling, support groups, meditation, regular physical activity, prayer groups, yoga, etc.

You might also have bad cholesterol, high triglycerides, high uric acid, high blood sugar, or high blood pressure. The lower abdomen will go down only when these things are normalized. A great benefit from the program is that even when you don't lose weight and measurements, it encourages in the normalization of these elements.

Hips and thighs: Fat cells in these areas are saturated with estrogen receptors, so any hormonal change (pregnancy, contraceptives, menopause) will affect them. The amount of fat in the diet impacts them also: excess fat in your diet may cause thighs and hips to increase.

If thighs are not going down, you are eating more fat than your body can burn off. Carefully check all the foods you're eating. Be obsessively critical of the way your meals are prepared. Most packaged food products, like instant soup, usually have lots of fats, and they are not good for this program.

If someone else cooks for you, confirm that they prepare food exactly as instructed in the program.

Stress will also affect our fat intake because when we are tense, the "phantom zone" increases, comfort foods loaded with fat become more appealing, and we eat more fat than we recognize.

Calves: Like the breasts, this circumference should change minimally. Calves can be a good reflection of how much muscle we have. When calves go down, it could mean that we are losing what we don't want to lose (muscle mass), and remember that this is the first step towards activating Starvation Mode.

By observing your body in the mirror and taking careful measurements on a regular basis, you can make sure you are reducing excess fat in the right places without generating Starvation Mode.

When you weigh and measure yourself, keep your cool no matter what result you get. Adverse changes in weight and measurements can cause you severe bouts of anguish, anger, and amnesia. Don't do that. It's not your body's fault that you punished it mercilessly for years with severe, ridiculous, and unhealthy diets.

In my day-to-day practice, I see two typical reactions:

The first is when a patient discovers he or she has lost weight and says, "Why did I lose weight if my diet was so disastrous?"

The second is when the patient's weight goes up, and he or she says, "I don't understand why this happened, I did the program perfectly."

To start with, nobody does a "perfect weight loss program." If you feel that way, you're deceiving yourself, which will not help at all.

Anyone who does the program diligently will sooner or later achieve results. If you find that weight has gone up, try to avoid selective amnesia about disordered eating during your program.

There are also events that make weight and volume go up even when you are doing the program "perfectly." The most important reason (and the one that should cause you the most concern) is a previous history of severe dieting and/or use of weight loss products.

Those who abandon a strict weight loss diet or discontinue weight loss pills run the risk of gaining weight as well as volume.

The menstrual period also causes weight gain, as well as a bloating belly and swollen mammary glands.

If you travel to hot climates, you can gain as much as two kilograms (4.4 pounds) due to fluid retention.

Other factors are high-salt diets and heavy drinking.

FOR DOCTORS AND NUTRITIONISTS

What would you say about a treatment that gives 95% recurrence, and that by the end of the treatment, the disease is on the average 20% worse than at the beginning? I totally agree with anyone who reaches the conclusion that traditional weight loss diets are useless.

There is no real hard, substantial evidence to continue using such treatment, and yet, people do it all the time!

No wonder doctors do not find interest in trying to help people lose excess weight with diets. It is frustrating and disheartening.

And it is no wonder that the general population is entirely disappointed with diets.

The solution must lie in changing the triggering events, and not on solving the sign, i.e. excess body weight.

I am not going to discuss all the research about causative mechanisms, but we all know that it does not have to do with a slow metabolism, lack of physical activity, and worse still, there is no clear evidence that it correlates with the amount of food that is overeaten. So why do we accumulate excess body fat?

The proportions theory is a much better way of explaining WHY the adipose system kicks into action. Let me explain:

Our body needs PROPORTIONALLY around 55% carbs, 30% fats, and 15% protein.

Protein is tightly regulated, and it does not fluctuate on the general population, be it based on animal or vegetable protein.

But fats and carbs are another story.

Regarding fats, population ingestion can range from 20% (typical diet eaten in Asia) to 55% (which is what the Inuit eat).

Now, my proportions theory states that if the distribution of macronutrients is severely altered, defense mechanisms kick in that increase the body's ability to store fat, i.e. Starvation Mode is activated.

The problem lies in the deviation macronutrients, and not on the excessive intake of any one of them.

Here's an example: let's say that someone is eating excessive quantities of carbohydrates, up to 70% of total intake, plus another 20% of protein. This leaves fat at around 10% of total caloric intake.

THIS NUTRIENT DISTRIBUTION (PROPORTION) WILL ACTIVATE THE BODY'S FAT STORING MECHANISMS.

The adipose system is not reacting to 70% carbs by storing fat.

It's responding to the extreme fat restriction activating Starvation Mode.

And here's the catch, Starvation Mode will not be evident until the person goes back to eating his usual percentage of dietary nutrients. If he continues with this nutrient distribution he will lose weight and volume!

Excess body fat does not appear while the person continues with the nutrient distribution of 70% carbs, 20% protein, and 10% fats.

This is what has thrown excess body fat treatment into total havoc: weight and volume are lost, but at the same time Starvation Mode is activated.

When the person goes back to eating a normal distribution of macronutrients, i.e. goes back to eating 30 to 40% (normal for the United States), his body accumulates excess body fat. Worse still, fat accumulates predominantly in the abdomen! Oh, and I forgot to mention that the amount of excess fat accumulated is not related to total caloric intake! It's related to the degree of Starvation Mode. That is why research studies cannot demonstrate a direct relationship between calories intake and weight gain.

When you shift from a 10% fat intake to a 35% fat intake, you accumulate excess body fat.

This is what happens to people who move from their native countries to the United States.

It's not the 35 to 40% of dietary fat eaten in the USA that causes accumulation of excess body fat, it is the shift from 10 or 20% to 35%.

That is why people end up 20% fatter after two years of following a strict diet.

Does this sound complicated? Well, it is!

Now, what about the new tendency to increase total dietary fat content to 60 or 70%? That would leave 15% protein and 15 to 25% carbs.

People will lose weight and volume on these diets, but again, Starvation Mode is triggered, and when people go back to eating NORMAL quantities of carbohydrates, excess body fat reappears, is increased by 20% AND ends up in the abdomen.

How did I reach these conclusions?

I decided to start creating diets with varying percentages of macronutrients. I would give my patients a diet for five whole days and then tell them they could eat whatever they wanted on the weekend.

If the distribution of macronutrients caused a rapid gain of weight and volume over the weekend, I would take that diet off my treatment arsenal.

What did I end up with after years of fine-tuning the macronutrient equation?

I ended up with the diets in this book and with a way to target fat loss.

You see, our job is not just to make people lose excess fat; we are here also to avoid it from coming back. Our work is not only to make the fever go away, but it is also to treat the underlying cause if we can.

We need to find a diet that does not cause people to regain weight when they go back to eating in a free-living condition.

And that diet should allow them to eat whatever they want on the weekends without regaining weight or volume.

I'm happy to say that I found a way, but it isn't easy.

How did we go wrong in treating excess body fat?

There is a HUGE ERROR that we have been making for years, which is that we are focusing on weight loss, and lately only to the loss of weight and volume.

It's not enough.

We cannot focus just on one or two circumferences, we must consider ALL OF THEM.

EVERY doctor knows that neither excess weight nor BMI clearly identifies excess body fat. It is the total percentage which is over 25% in men and 30% in women.

Why do we try to solve a problem with a measuring instrument that is non-specific?

As doctors, we must strive to obtain three things from someone who has excess body fat.

We need to reduce VOLUME as well as weight.

We need to make it go away it in the right places.

And we must make certain that weight and volume stay off when the person leaves his diet.

We have led the world astray, making people focus on an instrument that will not solve their problem and can even worsen it!

Imagine a doctor who tells his patients to take their body temperature to decide how many calories to eat depending on temperature readings. That would be strange, right?

Here is another complication: body weight is related to the activity of the adipose system as well as ALL THE OTHER SYSTEMS.

If the cardiovascular system fails, the weight will go up.

So why do we blame the adipose system when the weight goes up, and not the other systems?

And why do we tell our patients to restrict their food intake when we know that in the long run, it doesn't work?

Since the scale has neither specificity nor sensitivity regarding shifts of adipose tissue, I use a measuring tape to track the body's reaction to dietary manipulations.

For years, I measured my patient nude, or in light underwear. Therefore, I could identify the effect of varying percentages of nutrients on THE WHOLE BODY.

After years of observation, I discovered mathematical equations that I will share with you. These are the equations I use for targeted fat loss.

EQUATIONS FOR TARGETED FAT LOSS:

Fat loss on the upper third of abdomen + fat loss of cheeks

50% carbohydrate, 20% protein and 30% fat
High-quality protein, if possible, I use protein powder

Fat loss on middle third of abdomen

55% carbohydrates, 15% protein and 30% fat
An abundance of green leafy vegetables: juices, smoothies, etc.
As much variety as possible: pasta, rice, quinoa, tortilla, bagel, etc.

Fat loss on lower third of abdomen + fat loss on double chin

55% carbohydrates, 15% protein and 30% fat
35 grams or more of fiber, 50% or more of soluble fiber

Fat loss on hips, thighs, and arms

58% carbohydrates, 15% protein and 27% fat
Over 1,600 calories per day, ideally over 1,800 calories per day
The following foods excel in mobilizing gluteal fat: cold cooked corn, cold cooked potatoes, cold cooked beans, papaya, and any type of pasta.

Fat loss on shoulders

55% carbohydrates, 15% protein and 30% fat
At least 2,100 calories per day

Fat loss on chest

No balance is needed if food is eaten at specific hours.
The patient needs to eat something every 1 to 2 hours

Firmer breasts

52% carbohydrates, 15% protein and 33% fat
At least 1,800 calories per day
At least 3 ounces (90 grams) of pastry per day

Cellulite reduction

Very low content of saturated fat (less than 5% of total caloric value)
Over 60% vegetable protein
An abundance of green leafy vegetables: juices, smoothies, etc.

Firmer gluteus and larger calves

50% carbohydrates, 20% protein and 30% fat
10% animal fat and 20% vegetable fat
10% of protein from dairy products: cheese, whey protein, etc.
Over 1,800 calories per day

Cut body

53% carbohydrates, 20% protein and 27% fat
Over 2,000 calories per day
Meals are programmed every two hours
(This equation might cause a woman's breast to shrink but not sag)

I invite you to use these equations to create your own diets and try them on your patients. Results can be fascinating!

An easier solution is to buy the targeted fat loss diets that I have already created. You can find them at my Web page boliodiets

As you use these diets, you will gain experience in choosing the right one for each patient.

All my diets are based on low glycemic index foods, so you don't have to worry about giving them to your diabetic patients.

The next step is the most difficult one for us: to find out just how well our patients are following instructions!

You see, people believe that they apply ALL PROGRAMS TO PERFECTION.

This is impossible since patients are in a free-living environment, and between 20 and 40% of ingested calories will be eaten in the Phantom Zone (page 94).

The ONLY way to be SOMEWHAT confident that they are eating what they are supposed to, is to put them in a facility where all they must do is relax and eat what they are supposed to eat.

If there is anyone out there interested in creating a "fat farm" for my patients, I would be FASCINATED to do it. All we need is a vacation resort that wants to change people's lives.

When people do that, they can lose 5 to 7 dress sizes in less than a month! So much weight loss is possible that when they come back from their "vacations," not even family members recognize them!

A patient of mine did just that. I mentioned to her that taking vacations to diet would be the fastest way for her to lose weight. She did just that and went off to a coastal city with her childhood nanny. All she did that month was relax and enjoy her diet. When she came back, the security personnel who protected her workplace, and who had known her for years, did not recognize her and did not let her into her office! She was the personal secretary of a Secretary of State, hence the bodyguards.

Oh, and I didn't recognize her either. She came back with a spectacular figure and face that looked 30 years younger!

As a matter of fact, I want to be the first one to try out this "fat farm"! Obtain a cut abdomen and look 20 years younger, while eating every single imaginable dish? Oh, yeah, sign me up!

Ok, so back to reality, and to what we face daily:

YOU MUST TAKE MEASUREMENTS OR HAVE SOMEONE DO IT FOR YOU.

This is the only way to know what a person has done nutrition-wise in the previous weeks.

Where exactly you take your circumferences, it really doesn't matter if you do it consistently in the same areas. And of course, you must train your technician or nurse to be persistently accurate. I have already mentioned the areas I measure on pages 146 and 147.

Measuring a patient's circumferences is the ONLY way you will know whether he or she has eaten the way that you recommended or not.

Here's a rundown of what to consider if measurements go up:

Arm: they ate more fat than what was programmed. Instead of reducing fat from the menu, try increasing carbs.

Shoulder: they did not eat enough calories. Increase caloric value.

Breast: either they did not eat when they were supposed to, or in women, it could be that their breasts got bigger. Explain how important it is to eat when you are supposed to. If breasts went up and your female patients don't mind or are even happy, then ask them to continue with the plan! But if they are NOT HAPPY with breasts that are increasing, you must check with them just how many extra pastries they are indulging in!

Chest: they did not eat at the programmed hours. Insist that they eat when they are supposed to.

Upper third of abdomen: they need more protein in the diet. Consider going all the way up to 20% of calories from protein.

Middle third of abdomen: they did not eat enough vegetables, fruits, legumes, and/or they did not eat a balanced diet. Have them log their dietary intake.

Lower third of abdomen: they are living chronic stressful events. Increase soluble fiber through psyllium husk, artichoke and/or help them establish stress management techniques.

Hips: this one is a little tricky since hips can go up because gluteus muscles increase, because of gluteal fat increases, or both! Take a critical look at their glutes. Are they firm and toned? Then you are on track.

If on the contrary, they are sagging, it is because they are increasing gluteal fat. It also means that they are eating more fat than their body can metabolize. Instead of reducing fats, try increasing high carb foods.

Thighs: they ate more fat than what was programmed. Consider increasing the total carbs in their diet. By the way, if hips go up and thighs go down, it means that gluteus muscles are growing! This is my dream come true!

Calf: they are increasing muscle mass and retaining fluids. If it is due to fluid retention, it is usually because of low salt intake. Ask them to hike up salt in their diet. And don't worry about their blood pressure if they are losing weight and/or volume.

All my diets have less than 2 grams of salt per day, BUT ONLY IF SALT IS USED WHEN PREPARING MEALS. If they do not use salt when cooking meals, they will be eating a severely salt restricted diet and therefore severe shifts in body fluids will ensue, i.e., the weight will go up and down like crazy.

A word of caution: when people DO NOT lose weight and volume, they ALWAYS state that they followed the program perfectly. And in their minds, they did! But if measurements do not go down, they are not doing what they are supposed to.

When this happens, I say that the diet didn't work for them. Not because the diet doesn't work, but because it did not adapt to the patient's lifestyle.

This is the time you need to help your patients find a solution.

If they do not like vegetables, have them prepare veggie smoothies, or have them juice their vegetables. Or send them to cooking classes so that they can learn how to cook tasty vegetable dishes. It's not that they don't like veggies; they just don't know how to make them taste great!

In my daily practice, I find the following impediments for loss of volume:

Fear of food (this is number one)

Fear of the scale (this is number two)

Total ignorance of nutrition

Previous low carb dieting

Previous extremely low-calorie dieting

Plateau

Previous major surgeries: tonsillectomy, gallbladder removal, C-section, appendectomy, hysterectomy, etc.

Non-logical expectations

Lack of time

Boredom

A highly stressful life

Insomnia

Impaired micro-biota

Leaky Gut

Then there is another event that has baffled me for years:

If patients have any altered lab work, such as high LDL cholesterol, high A1C, low hemoglobin, etc., they will not lose weight, or they will lose it very slowly until those parameters are normalized.

Fortunately, all my diets help people normalize their altered lab work. I am delighted with these results, but on the other hand, I am most unhappy with the following: I created a weight loss program that could care less about fast weight loss. My programs work first on helping the body get healthy, and only afterward will my diets cause a rapid loss of weight and inches. Ugh!

Can you imagine my frustration?

There is another reason for the lack of weight loss, and to explain it, I will tell you a story about one patient.

A patient who had blood in his urine came to see me, not for weight loss, but to find out if my diet could help him eliminate blood from his urine. He had been thoroughly checked for causative factors, but all his studies had come back negative. This did not mean that he did not have severe disease of the urinary tract, it just said that nothing had come out positive. Ugh again!

I told him that I had seen fascinating cases of people who reversed many problems, including cancer when on my diet and that even though his doctors did not have a definite diagnosis for his bloody urine, the program would not hurt him.

After one month on his diet, the blood in his urine disappeared. This made both of us extremely happy! And that was more than enough reason for him to continue with the diet.

I did explain to him that even though blood had disappeared, he needed to continue to be checked by his doctor to rule out any severe problem such as cancer or tuberculosis.

Here is the interesting part: he did not lose any weight or volume! But he was so happy with the results that he turned the diet into his personal lifestyle, not for weight loss, since he was not losing anything, but because his urine studies had come out normal.

Six months later he came back to see me, utterly terrified because he had lost TEN POUNDS IN ONE WEEK.

He knew that blood in the urine could be a sign of cancer and he was horrified to consider this possibility.

I took measurements, sent him to be checked by his nephrologist, and asked him to come back in a week to recheck measurements.

A week later he had lost 5 MORE POUNDS, but happily, his calf had maintained the same circumference, which led me to believe that he was only losing excess body fat and not muscle mass.

And for someone to lose only excess body fat with an ad-libitum diet at such a fast rate, it is almost impossible for him to have any underlying disease.

So, I told him not to worry, and to wait for study results, which would most probably be normal.

And they were! There was no blood in urine, and there was no cancer!

This is an anecdotal case, but many of my patients have gone through similar situations: they maintain weight and volume week after week, and after months of waiting, suddenly start losing excess body fat at spectacular rates.

Why is it that some people do not initially lose weight and volume with a balanced diet? What underlying issue could hinder loss of excess body fat? Most of the time, I never find out.

And not everyone loses volume with this diet. Around 80% of my patients lose excess body fat, while the other 20% do not. Out of that 20%, 5% will gain weight and inches.

Why is it that some people don't ever lose volume, or even gain some? Maybe tomorrow we will know. And obviously, the more we know about what makes our body accumulate excess body fat, the more efficient we will be in treating it.

I find this more fascinating than anguishing. Truthfully, the adipose system is a territory that we are just barely beginning to explore!

Here is another phenomenon that fascinates me: I have treated patients who reversed mild kidney damage due to diabetes. And diabetic patients who I treated have lived with their blood glucose at normal levels for years. You can include my mother and other family members on that list.

There is another phenomenon that my fellow doctors will love. The program helps control diabetes mellitus, high blood pressure, low HDL, high LDL, high sedimentation rate, fatty liver, asthma, lupus, cancer, COPD, chronic fatigue, fibroids, fibromyalgia, rheumatoid arthritis, insomnia, depression, anger, diminished ability to fight off infections, brain fog, menstrual cramps, infertility, low libido, hair loss, gray hair, acne and many other problems.

How can one diet affect so many different systems?

It doesn't. I believe that the diet is only helping the body heal itself.

But then, it is a wonderful way to help our patients recover from whatever they are going through.

Now, about people who do not lose weight or even gain some:

My recommendation for these cases is to apply what I call the "concentration camp protocol" since not one single person who survived concentration camps came out obese.

I will give them the Simeons protocol with Human Chorionic Gonadotropin (HCG) because this program gives results that are like my diets, i.e. when done correctly, the HCG diet causes minimal loss of structural fat.

But after the Simeons diet, they must go back to eating an ad libitum meal.

A word on supplements: keep away from them.

Since I measure patients as well as weigh them, I can state that I have not found one single supplement, medication or combination that I have found useful in long-term body fat mobilization.

It is even worse than that. Since patients feel that "the pill" is enough, they do not follow the program, and when I check results, I find that they gained volume even when weight was lost.

There is one combination that I used 37 years ago with extraordinary success: naloxone plus fenfluramine. I would have my patients inject themselves naloxone and at the same time take fenfluramine. This combination generated spectacular results, and it was common to see people lose 5 to 7 dress sizes in a month!

This is equivalent to a loss of anywhere from 30 to 40 pounds of body fat. It is supposed to be impossible, but since I didn't know that it was impossible, I never even considered publishing it!

By the way, I used this combination 15 years before the Phen/Fen craze.

But neither naloxone, nor fenfluramine, nor any other medication will teach people to eat in a balanced manner, i.e., it is useless for long-term weight control.

We can now use nasal naltrexone but at a ridiculous cost. I prefer to use HCG.

There are many more things that I could write about in relation to my 37 plus years of treating excess body fat, but it would probably not add too much more to what you have already read. So, let's wrap it up.

CONCLUSIONS:

We are faced with a problem that has been poorly managed, and the main reason for this is everyone's obsession with weight loss when weight loss is entirely useless.

When we finally view the fat cell as a system, and not as a problem, then we will become more skillful at treating it.

There is much to do:

I would love to have a national average of multiple body circumferences for every age, gender, weight, and race.

I would love for all centers that treat excess body fat to report their results in circumferences as well as weight.

I would love to hear from all my fellow doctors as to how their diabetic patients responded to my program. Did I mention that I have seen diabetic nephropathy reverted in very disciplined patients?

We also need to understand how and why modifying macronutrients impact body fat in such different ways.

And then all sorts of questions arise:

Is the hip reducing diet working because estrogen levels are diminished, or for another reason?

Can we manipulate fat mobilization in such a way that we can help the body heal other organs?

I find it all fascinating.

And I hope that I can count on your support with this new concept of the adipose system, and above all, on treating patients with an ad libitum balanced diet.

And finally, I do hope that I will see in my lifetime the tendency of obesity to revert towards normal bodies!

Happy hunting!

Made in the USA
Middletown, DE
18 February 2018